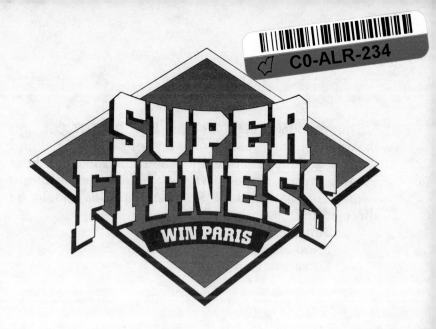

SUPER FITNESS
WIN PARIS

PRICE/STERN/SLOAN
Publishers, Inc., Los Angeles
1978

The products mentioned in SUPER FITNESS are brand names marketed by the author's company, Super Fitness of America. Similar products, especially those dealing with nutrition, are available under different names in retail outlets. Product inquiries should be directed to:

Super Fitness of America
23650 Hawthorne Boulevard
Torrance, California 90505

Front Cover — Author Win Paris and his wife, Tami Paris, exercising on a California beach.
Design and Photography by Francis Morgan

This Book, My Philosophy of Super Fitness, is dedicated to five of the many hundreds of people who helped create it:

My wife, Tami, who inspired DISCIPLINE

My Mother, who inspired LOVE

Dr. Laurence Morehouse, PH.D., UCLA, whose book, TOTAL FITNESS inspired me to write this book

Dr. Donald T. Handy, UCLA, who inspired UNDERSTANDING

Dr. Valerie Hunt, UCLA, who inspired WISDOM

Super Fitness Creed

MY

ONLY

LIMITATIONS

ARE

ME!

SUPER THOUGHTS

+

SUPER ATTITUDE

+

SUPER PRAYER

+

SUPER ACTION

+

SUPER NUTRITION

+

SUPER EXERCISE

=

SUPER

ME!

ABOUT THE AUTHOR

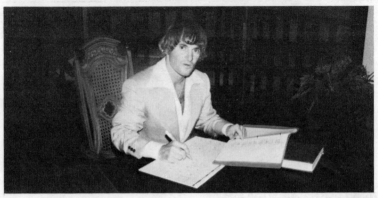

Since winning the First Junior Mr. L.A. Contest at the age of 20, Win Paris has been involved in a wide variety of fitness related activities including corrective and physical therapy, physical education, the health spa industry, and fitness education on national TV.

While a student at UCLA, he won the Southern Pacific Lightweight Wrestling Championship and also competed in gymnastics. He received Bachelor of Science and Master of Science degrees in the therapeutic aspects of Physical Education from UCLA, and a Certified Corrective Physical Therapy Certificate from UCLA. From USC he qualified as a Registered Physical Therapist. He has also completed all course requirements for a Ph.D.

While at UCLA, he was elected to Phi Epsilon Kappa and Phi Delta Kappa, national honorary scholastic societies in Physical Education and Education, respectively.

Win taught corrective physical education in the Los Angeles schools for four years and during this time he became the National Bench Press champion in the lightweight division with a 320-pound official press.

At the age of 30, he founded and directed the Physician's Physical Therapy Service which operated 12 physical therapy departments for hospitals, orthopedic surgeons, medical groups and convalescent hospitals in Southern California.

In 1968, he established the popular Jack La Lanne Health Spas and served as president of La Lanne-Paris, Inc. Four years later he founded that company's highly successful Nutritional Education Division. He is credited with the creation of the Fitness Educator concept.

Today, Win, as president and founder of Super Fitness of America, is recognized as the nation's Number One Fitness Educator.

CONTENTS

STEP FOUR — PART ONE
Super Exercise

STEP FOUR — PART TWO
Super Nutrition

INTRODUCTION

SUPER FITNESS begins in your MIND!
YOUR MIND CONTROLS YOUR MOUTH!
YOUR MIND CONTROLS YOUR BODY!
YOUR MIND CONTROLS YOUR DESTINY ON EARTH!

Thus, SUPER FITNESS begins with a super state of mind and a super state of mind begins with a SUPER SPIRITUAL EXPERIENCE.

You can become SUPER FIT and enjoy a SUPER LIFE by:

1. Developing a SUPER SPIRIT which continually helps you to triumph over YOURSELF.

2. Developing a SUPER MIND by using it as much as possible and controlling the quality of your thoughts.

3. Maintaining a pleasing, positive SUPER AT-TITUDE.

4. Developing SUPER FITNESS OF YOUR BODY by eating slowly and eating small quantities of fresh pure food as close to its natural state as possible, plus natural food supplements, while continually increasing your physical activity.

You are starting your exciting new SUPER FITNESS life RIGHT NOW!

CONGRATULATIONS!

YOU ARE ON YOUR WAY TO SUPER FITNESS AND THE SUPER LIVING WHICH SUPER FITNESS MAKES POSSIBLE.

Step One

Super Fitness

This may be the only section on SUPER FITNESS to drag you down.

My purpose in life is to INSPIRE, EDUCATE and ACTIVATE my fellow man toward a Super Life.

But you must know that I am one of you.

I am human, too.

Whatever blessing of Super Spirit, mind and body I have, I had to earn.

The battle is not over; super living requires a daily battle for victory over yourself.

You, too, can and will triumph over yourself and enjoy SUPER LIVING.

Just put into practice the message in this book.

DO IT!

For there was a day when I was devoid of spirit.

I was empty.

Life was chaos.

My purpose in life was confusion.

I wandered, lost.

I had no idea where to go or what to do.

I cried,

I sighed.

I prayed.

I was so depressed, obsessed and exhausted by negative thoughts of poverty that I could not get out of bed until almost noon after trying to go to sleep 12 hours earlier.

At times the nerves in my body tingled with tremors as if they were live wires.

I was exhausted.

I consulted psychiatrists, took tranquilizers and grabbed at every straw that held out even the slightest hope for mental-emotional tranquility.

I visited a score of churches trying to fill my emptiness.

I was so poor that I had to accept my mother's 30 year-old carpet and sofa so I could have some furniture in my tiny apartment.

I felt like a dog that had become covered with fleas and I didn't have the energy to kill them.

My world was confined to work and bed.

My friends were few.

I'll never forget one summer when I went to the state office of employment.

As a corrective Physical Education teacher, I had three months vacation and I needed to earn some extra money to live.

What a feeling of dejection, self-pity and lack of esteem to stand in line looking for work and then be told that I didn't have the qualifications for any of the routine jobs available.

Life seemed so hopeless.

I remember how I cried in emptiness in front of my mother when I was feeling especially sorry for myself.

Even though I knew I was debasing myself, I couldn't hold back the tears which flooded forth from my emotionally wracked body.

Still another time I was so depressed that I was afraid to see anyone I knew, afraid that they would see my fear and weakness and laugh at the defeated attitude which dominated my mind.

I was so negative and down that I felt I couldn't hide my innermost feelings no matter how hard I tried.

For almost six months I was so exhausted emotionally and physically that all I could do was lie around the house.

I felt like a vegetable.

I did not realize the incredible power of thought.

Because I thought like a vegetable, I became like a vegetable.

My physical appearance mirrored the mental condition I was in.

I put on weight.

I got so fat that I wore baggy clothes to hide the bulges.

I wouldn't get into a bathing suit for fear someone would make a remark about my "potbelly."

But, there was no hiding my fat face and double chins.

I could not fool myself and, unfortunately, I couldn't control my mouth.

I was a glutton seeking escape in feasting.

I paid for it with my "potbelly," my appearance and my pride.

LOST.
BROKE.
SPIRITUALLY EMPTY.
GOAL-LESS
WEAK.
HOPELESS.

Then I remembered the Bible and the Book of Proverbs.

It had been of great solace to me before.

Why hadn't I remembered it now?

I began to read it.

The Bible gave me what I needed:

A SPIRITUAL base to life.

And on that base, I began to build.

My spiritual fitness began to grow.

My attitude improved, as did my mental and physical fitness.

I usually don't discuss this phase of my life, but I want to share it with you so that you will see that I have been where you have been or may be right now!

And I am where you are going!

You are on your way to a wondrous new life with Super Fitness of your spirit, mind, attitude and body.

A mind vigorous to think and grow.

An attitude that helps you to turn problems into opportunities!

A body surging with energy.

A human whose destiny is charted with divine guidance!

The most dramatic turning point came one evening when I was on my knees and I saw a bright, full moon.

I was in an environment worse than Hell, to put it mildly.

That moon, so pure and clear and real, inspired me.

For I knew that only God could create such a wondrous sight.

I WAS BORN ANEW!

And that's why I know YOU can be born anew!

Just by getting one spark of inspiration and holding one positive thought in your mind, YOU ARE DOING IT!

YOU ARE A WINNER IF YOU THINK YOU ARE!

Repeat to yourself:

"I AM A SUPER WINNER!"

Repeat it 100 times a day for one full week.

Don't think about it . . . DO IT!

IT WORKS!

YOU ARE A SUPER WINNER!

Write me a letter and tell me you are REBORN!

Tell me you are a SUPER WINNER!

Do it RIGHT NOW!

I want to hear from you.

Write to: WIN PARIS, c/o Price/Stern/Sloan Publishers, Inc., 410 N. La Cienega Blvd., Los Angeles, CA 90048.

DO IT NOW!

CONGRATULATIONS!

The Nitty Gritty of Super Fitness:
G-Complex

Let's get down to the nitty-gritty.

The heart of how to attain SUPER FITNESS.

The secret is simple:

Get turned on, get inspired, get angry at yourself!

Set self-improvement goals, as outlined in step 4 of this book.

Say to yourself, "I know how great I'm going to look if I lose that extra ten or twenty or thirty pounds."

"My double chin will disappear and this ugly fat around my waist will evaporate."

"I will look ten years younger."

"All my friends and even my family will admire me for having the determination, the fortitude and the guts to lose that ugly flab."

The key is simple:

Get turned on, determined, psyched up, whatever you want to call it — BUT DO IT NOW!

You slob (I'm trying to get you angry at yourself!).

You can be a winner!

Who said you had to be a loser?

It was YOU!

You can discard all the messages that made you think you were a loser.

You can be renewed.

First control your mind.

Then control your mouth!

Losing that extra 10 or 20 pounds will give you a storehouse of super energy.

You will save your heart from pumping gallons of blood for the pounds of fat that you are overweight!

You will save your body the two miles of extra capillaries needed to feed each extra 10 pounds of fat that you are overweight!

You're going to look super-trim and super-sexy!

You're going to save your life!

FAT IS FATAL!

If you are 30 percent over your normal weight, you have increased your chances by 40 percent for an early death over a person of normal bodyweight.

A TIP FROM THE NATIONAL HEART ASSOCIATION — FAT KILLS!

As far as I'm concerned, obesity is the Number One health problem in the United States today.

Over 50 million Americans are overweight!

Just plain fat!

You owe it to your children to lose that fat before it kills you and deprives them of a father or a mother or a grandparent.

Dante's "Inferno" refers to gluttons who are sentenced to eternal damnation for being fat.

The Bible says in Proverbs 23: "For the Drunkard and the Glutton Shall Come to Poverty."

Sir Richard Burton said, "Gluttony is the source of all of our infirmities and the fountain of all our diseases."

I hope you realize by now that I am trying to back you into a corner. I am pushing you to the edge of a cliff.

You can either be a lazy loser and jump off the cliff and take the easy way out, or you can get mad at me or yourself or anyone else, and change for the better!

CHARGE at life and conquer it with your great new vibrant looks and your dynamic new super energy!

Say to yourself ONE HUNDRED times each morning and evening:

"I am going to control my mind."

"I am going to lose that extra fat fast by a combination of intelligent eating and increased physical activity."

"My magic ingredient is D I S C I P L I N E!"

"I have it! I'm going to keep it and I'm going to lead a wondrously healthy happy SUPER NEW LIFE starting right now!

"I am going to tranquilize with exercise and throw away the pills."

"I am going to throw the garbage out of my kitchen!"

"I AM A SUPER WINNER!"

"I am glad to be alive AND I AM GOING TO LIVE THE RADIANT NEW LIFE I WAS INTENDED TO LIVE IN THE FIRST PLACE!"

Keep a picture of the trim new you in your mind.

See yourself looking fantastic, wearing the clothes you've always wanted to wear.

See yourself feeling the new vibrant super energy flowing through your body.

See it giving you the energy to work harder and play harder and be a better lover and a better person.

YOU WILL BECOME WHAT YOU THINK ABOUT.

Say to yourself:

"I AM SUPER FIT!"

YOU ARE SUPER FIT!

Step Two

Super Mental Fitness

Victory Over Yourself

The true battlefield which decides your triumph or defeat in your achieving SUPER FITNESS lies within your mind!

You CAN become master of your fate.

You ARE master of your fate.

The first thing to do is LOOK IN THE MIRROR!

Stare at your eyes.

Say to yourself:

"I will eat small portions of fresh natural food!"

"I will be physically active each and every day!"

"I will keep a pleasant positive attitude toward all!"

"I will fight for and get a trim, attractive and healthy waistline!"

"I will win the battle of the bulge!"

"I will triumph over myself!"

"I will triumph over life!"

"I will not be dependent upon drugs, tranquilizers, uppers, downers, shots or pills!"

"I will not drain the emotions of others!"

"I will not be a parasite!"

"I will make my life exciting and triumphant!"

"I will plan my life. I will work my plan!"

"I will live anew!"

"I AM LIVING ANEW!"

"From this moment on, I will begin to achieve victory over my greatest enemy: MYSELF!"

REMEMBER:

"WE SQUANDER HEALTH IN SEARCH OF WEALTH
WE SCHEME AND TOIL AND SAVE,
THEN SQUANDER WEALTH IN SEARCH OF HEALTH
AND ALL WE GET IS A GRAVE.
WE LIVE AND BOAST OF WHAT WE OWN,
WE DIE
AND ONLY GET A STONE!"

Anonymous

Your Wondrous Mind

If you practice my philosophy of SUPER FITNESS, you will feel fantastic!

I'm not just saying words, I mean it.

Right now, I feel as if I could jump up and fly!

It's a sort of hyper-state you get in your mind.

You feel like flying!

Many of you have had it before.

What you think about all day, you become.

If you think you're a loser, you will be a loser.

If you think you're a winner, you will become a winner.

YOU BECOME WHAT YOU THINK ABOUT MOST!

Although I am a corrective therapist, a physical therapist, a physical education teacher and a 30-year student of nutrition and exercise, I firmly believe that the THOUGHTS YOU PUT IN YOUR MIND ARE MORE IMPORTANT THAN THE FOOD YOU PUT IN YOUR BODY!

UNHEALTHY THOUGHTS WILL POISON YOUR MIND.

FROM THIS DAY FORWARD, ELIMINATE ALL UN-HEALTHY THOUGHTS FROM YOUR MIND.

Why eat healthy foods, exercise, wear fancy clothes, and then think negative destructive thoughts?

Set a goal in your mind of how you want to look, the type of mind you want to develop, the type of person you want to become. HOLD THIS VISION as clearly as a photograph in your mind.

Many people will try to discourage you because they are jealous and don't know where they are going.

But you have a goal in your mind!

And, you can reach it!

You only have to think and work toward your positive goal. By a positive goal, I don't mean a phony phrase such as "I will be happy all day."

You must set up a positive specific program for the person you want to become and work toward becoming that person.

You should not be content with mediocrity.

It's a real bore, and life should not be a bore.

It's super exciting!

So make that goal.

Make it right now!

Think super thoughts from now on.

Super, healthy thoughts!

Control your mind and your life.

You are only using a small percentage of your brain.

The power of the brain, relatively speaking, is unlimited.

Most people don't take the time to do creative thinking.

Start growing mentally today!

Don't be surprised if your goal keeps changing.

It won't be the goal alone that is changing.

As you grow and reach your goal, you will change and your dreams and aspirations will grow with you.

Have goals for every day, every week, every month and every year of your life.

If you do not have goals in life, you'll be like a ship sailing in the ocean without any idea of where it is going.

No matter what your profession, or how much money you have or whether you are married, single, masculine or feminine, you must have goals.

You must control your life!

You must not let others push you in a multitiude of directions.

You must set goals for yourself and get going.

GET OFF YOUR REAR AND GET INTO GEAR!

Get your life rolling!

Don't procrastinate!

I used to be the worst procrastinator in the world.

Once you get in motion, it's hard to stop.

All of a sudden you become a Doer!

Your motto should be "DO IT NOW."

Point yourself in the right direction.

Don't just think about doing it, DO IT!

You develop capabilities to analyze every situation because each situation is different.

Think and then act!

Become a POSITIVE THINKER and POSITIVE DOER!

Here is a formula to improve your thinking, your body and your life.

It's called Paris' I.D.E.A. FORMULA for SUPER FITNESS, which I created when I opened my first medical health club in Torrance, California, in 1965.

I.D.E.A. FORMULA

"I" IS FOR INSPIRATION

The first thing you must do to change your life into one of SUPER FITNESS is to be inspired.

Always remember, you can reach your SUPER FITNESS goals.

"D" IS FOR DESIRE.

Next, create a desire within yourself.

I like to look at people and see their X-factors.

Physically, do they have big rears and fat thighs?

Do they have potbellies?

Bustlines sagging and hanging?

Negative attitudes?

Flabby arms?

Is their hair short and stringy and falling apart? Cracked fingernails? Are they overweight?

Remember, visualize daily in your mind how you will look and feel. Build your desire and light your internal fire to become the super looking person you want to be.

"E" IS FOR EDUCATION

Get educated!

Become an avid reader of books on nutrition, exercise, physiology and self-improvement.

Become educated on how to attain SUPER FITNESS.

Make it a hobby to study about your mind, body, nutrition and exercise.

"A" IS FOR ACTION

Action separates the winners from the losers.

When I taught corrective physical education, the biggest gap was between theory and practice.

ACTIONS speak louder than words.

You need action to reach your goal!!

Remember, there is only one person who can set a limit for you.

That person is YOU!

To repeat, be a positive Thinker AND a positive Doer.

Your Mind Controls Your Body
Your Body Reflects Your Mind

Think about those two sentences.

If you are fat, it is because you are uneducated and/or undisciplined in regard to exercise and nutrition. (These statements, in my opinion, cover 95 percent of all people. Don't look for other reasons for being fat!).

By uneducated, I mean you have not learned about the fundamentals of your mind, nutrition and exercise in order to control your body fat.

By undisciplined, I mean that as far as your nutritional and physical activities are concerned, you know how much to eat, what to eat, how to exercise, BUT YOU JUST DON'T DO IT because you are lazy and lack DISCIPLINE.

But you cannot fool your body!

If you eat junk your body becomes JUNKY!

If you do not get enough physical activity, your body will reflect this to an exact degree in terms of strength, circulation, endurance, flexibility, beauty, appearance, etc., etc.

You must EARN a beautiful appearance.

The formula is simple.
INSPIRATION + DESIRE
  +
EDUCATION
  +
ACTIVATION = RESULTS!
Remember, there is no substitute for positive action.

My third job is to activate you.

That's why I have modified Norman Vincent Peale's concept of "The Power of Positive Thinking" to my concept of "POSITIVE ACTION," based on the following formula:

POSITIVE THOUGHT + POSITIVE ACTION = RESULTS!

Let's call it "The Paris Concept of Positive Action!"

I called it by my name out of pride of creativity, plus identification, so that people who heard of this concept and needed help in understanding and applying it to their lives could come to me for help.

Positive action, in relation to nutrition and physical activity, will produce a beautiful, healthy, efficient body, no matter how bad you look or feel.

I repeat, YOUR BODY REFLECTS YOUR MIND.

My goal is to inspire and educate your mind and activate your body.

If you follow the principles of thought, nutrition and physical activity in this book, your wildest dreams about how you want to look, feel and live will come true!

You will have new energy and stamina.

You will add a sparkle to your eyes, a spring to your step and a joy to your heart!

Remember, YOUR BODY REFLECTS YOUR MIND.

When you violate sound principles of thought, nutrition and physical activity, you are cheating only one person in the world:YOU!

So join me on a new path of life.

Be an upper, not a downer.

A winner, not a loser.

Control your mind, and your body.

Paint on your wall, or carve on your door, or draw a sign with the following words in capital letters: DO IT NOW! CAPITAL DO, CAPITAL IT, CAPITAL NOW, with a big exclamation point! DO IT NOW!

Let's get down to specifics.

Your mind controls how your body looks.

I recently went into the kitchen of an acquaintance, looked into the well-stocked refrigerator and saw only one thing that I would eat!

That was celery. The rest was chocolate syrup, processed cheese, pickles and you name a foodless food and it was there!

This person was literally living on processed and synthetic food.

It was a wonder how that family managed to survive!

However, Mother Nature is very tolerant.

She does not take your life quickly when your body is poorly nourished.

IT IS A SLOW process!

But the quality of your life does suffer.

I immediately suggested to the family above, and I suggest to you, a book on nutrition, such as Linda Clark's excellent one, "Stay Younger Longer."

Read the Labels on the food packages and don't eat anything with chemical additives.

EAT FRESH FOOD.

One of the key words to good nutrition is FRESH.

When I lived in Europe in 1955, many Europeans did not have refrigerators and, it proved very advantageous.

The lack of refrigeration made them healthier because they were eating fresh food, which they bought daily at the market.

Food starts to die as soon as it's picked!

So the less time from the field to your table, the better.

If you eat dead foods you are going to have, relatively speaking, a dead body!

If you eat junk foods, you're going to have a junky body!

But if you want a vivacious body that is alive and

glowing with umph and charisma, sexual appeal, allure and vitality, you must eat fresh, alive foods.

This is not really complicated; it's just common sense.

If you eat food that is alive, it is transformed in your body into your body and you will truly become more alive.

For the rest of your life, from this day forward, I want you to read labels on the foods you buy and eat as many fresh foods in their natural state as possible.

The poisons you eat in foods that have preservatives, in my opinion, build up over the years and may some day even prove to be a major source of cancer.

The other way your mind controls your body is in what you do.

If you are lazy and basically inactive, your body reflects the inactivity.

Your muscles lose their tone and start sagging.

Your circulation gets sluggish and, in general, you become lazier and weaker.

You look lazy, you feel lazy and you are lazy!

One of the secrets for a SUPER LIFE is to stay physically active.

Right now, I'd like to address office workers.

You have a rough job!

Sitting eight hours a day is one of the worst things you can do to your body and your health.

If nature had intended you to sit all day, you would have been born with a chair attached to your rear!

When you are sitting, typing, taking dictation, or answering phones, tension is building up in your body.

Secretaries, especially, build up tension in their upper backs, necks and shoulders because as they hold up their arms stress is forced on the shoulder muscles and surrounding musculature.

You build tension around the shoulder girdle and these tight muscles cut off circulation.

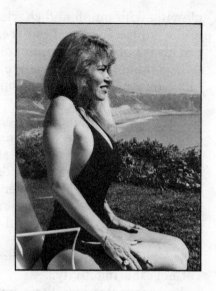

The muscles constrict against the blood vessels and the smooth pliable muscle fills with fibrous tissues due to decreased circulation.

Your muscles become tender and painful. When you make a sudden movement at night or turn your head, this tissue may tear painfully.

You avoid the pain by not moving and it becomes a vicious cycle.

If you sit all day in an office, I recommend that you do about five shoulder shrugs an hour, first shrugging up, forward and down and then up, backward and down.

Also perform the hug and squeeze for your upper back. Then move your elbows back and squeeze your shoulders together. Perform this five times each hour.

So now you can understand that your body is a combination of what you think, eat and do.

Your mind controls the activity that affects your body.

Your mind controls what you eat, what you do and therefore your appearance.

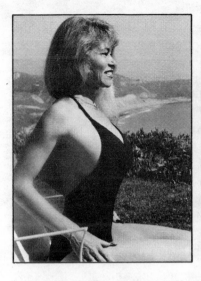 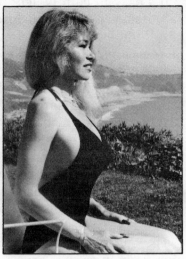

Some people think, "I was born to be fat."
Others think, "I was born to be skinny."
A basic concept of physiological psychology is that a skinny person can gain weight or a fat person can lose weight by understanding nutrition and exercise.

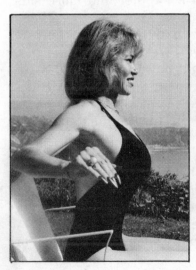 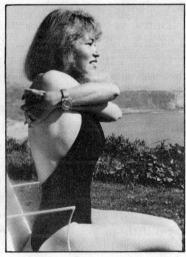

It's easy to gain weight.

A heavy person can lose weight if he controls his mind, understands and practices sound nutrition, and increases physical activity.

The point I am making is that your mind controls not only your destiny and the happiness of your life but also controls your appearance.

When you see a sharp looking man with a trim waist and a good body, you know he has practiced discipline to keep physcially active.

When you see a lady with a firm, trim figure, you can bet she has had to work for it.

The only thing you are born with is the raw material.

The rest is up to YOU!

The earlier in life your children learn this, the happier their lives will be.

They must EARN their health and appearance.

Educators have long known that a child's physical appearance in school is a great factor in the child's popularity.

So, if you teach children about SUPER FITNESS, you will be starting them off to a happier and more successful life.

Don't you wish someone had shown you how to become SUPER FIT when you were a child?

I would like to suggest right now, and every day for the rest of your life, that you spend 30 minutes daily developing your mind.

Read an educational or an inspirational book 15 minutes in the morning and 15 minutes in the evening.

It should be a book that stimulates your mind.

If you stop to think about it, a large part of your day is spent doing routine work.

It doesn't require much creative thinking to get out of bed, brush your teeth, drive to work, or watch TV.

So little of your day is actually spent doing critical or creative thinking.

If you don't spend at least a half hour a day doing this kind of thinking, instead of routine thinking, there is no way your mind and your life are going to become creative and exciting.

My first emphasis in life is on the spirit.

My second emphasis is your mind which you should develop through reading, thinking, evaluating, and planning, at least a half hour a day.

The Power of Thought

As you go about your daily living, accentuate the super constructive thoughts and eliminate the destructive. It's a must for SUPER MENTAL FITNESS!

I've listed some thoughts both constructive and destructive to help alert your senses. Add some of your own to the list.

SUPER CONSTRUCTIVE THOUGHTS	SUPER DESTRUCTIVE THOUGHTS
LOVE	FEAR
HOPE	JEALOUSY
FAITH	HATRED
WEALTH	REVENGE
DESIRE	DECEIT
WILL	FAILURE
COURAGE	SICKNESS
TRIUMPH	IMPOSSIBILITY
CONVICTION	POVERTY
BEAUTY	GREED
GOODNESS	DESPAIR
FRIENDSHIP	LONELINESS
POSITIVENESS	SUSPICION
HAPPINESS	DOUBT
LAUGHTER	UGLINESS
TRUST	ANGER
HEALTH	SORROW
SUCCESS	DEATH

Read, Read, Read

The wisdom of the ages is in books.

The books you read can transport you out of a dull world into every exciting place on earth.

Books can help you become friends with great people and great minds.

Books can help you become an expert in any field.

Since it is inevitable that we become what we think, I recommend you read and think about the wisdom contained in the autobiographies of such great people as CHURCHILL, GANDHI, LINCOLN, JEFFERSON, FRANKLIN.

Learn from the experience of others.

We know history and life are closely linked so it's to our advantage to learn from the past.

I would like to suggest again that you read for at least 30 minutes a day.

Read articles and/or books which will help complement you and your goals.

INVEST IN YOURSELF.

INVEST IN YOUR MIND.

Reading is an essential part of SUPER FITNESS because it EXERCISES YOUR BRAIN.

The more you exercise your brain, the stronger and better those millions of brain cells will become. The stronger they become, THE BETTER YOU WILL BECOME.

You'll be able to think accurately.

You'll become more of a leader and less of a follower.

Your life will become more interesting.

You will become more interesting.

You will learn more.

You will grow more as a person.

Reading will help you rise above the person who neglects his mind and brain.

Don't forget, your brain is the most powerful organ in your body.

USE IT OR LOSE IT!

It is stated in the Proverbs of the Bible . . .

"Get wisdom, get understanding . . ."

"Forsake her not and she will preserve thee . . ."

"And the years of thy life shall be many." (Prov. 4, Verse 5,6)

Ten Commandments
of Positive Action for Super
Mental Fitness

(1) Give your mind super daily activity for super development.

(2) Be an active thinker not a passive watcher.

(3) Read an educational or inspirational book for at least 30 minutes a day.

(4) Meditate upon the thoughts of great people.

(5) Tell yourself continually that you have a great mind and it will become even greater.

(6) Seek friends who have healthy strong minds.

(7) Practice Super Nutrition to nourish your brain to the optimum.

(8) Practice Super Exercise daily. Your mind and body are one. The health and strength of your body affects the health and strength of your brain.

(9) Control your mind and its thoughts, and concentrate especially on the spiritual basis of life each morning and evening.

(10) Set Mental goals for yourself each month. Make a calendar of events which will stimulate your brain into thinking new and great thoughts.

Step Three

Super Pleasing
Positive Attitude

Now, let's discuss the importance of a super pleasing positive attitude.

To me it's a matter of life and death.

If you're an optimist enjoying a bright sunny day, you're thankful for such a beautiful day.

A pessimist looks at a sunny day and says tomorrow it will probably rain!

No matter what is happening in life, look for the good things because there are always good and bad sides.

My attitude is, if you find a problem — SOLVE IT!

Think of a problem as an exciting challenge.

In fact, I get excited and say to myself, "Oh boy, this is something I will solve!"

If you have a positive attitude, your life becomes completely different.

Life becomes an exciting challenge.

Your mind creates the reality.

If you look for the good things in life, life is good.

If you are happy — you make other people happy.

If you're a downer or a pessimist you drag everybody else down around you.

There are people who have such pleasing positive attitudes they draw people, as flies are drawn to honey. People won't let them go and this is the person you want to be.

You want a lot of friends and you want people to like and love you.

Pessimistic people are actually filled with negative charges that repel people.

There are some people who call you on the phone or knock on your door and you just want to run and hide.

You don't want to be around them.

I want you to start realizing how important your attitude is.

Develop a super pleasing and positive attitude.

Be a realist.

Identify the problems.

Think of them as challenges and solve them.

First develop a pleasing attitude and DISCARD ALL UNHEALTHY THOUGHTS IN YOUR MIND.

If you have unhealthy thoughts and a negative attitude, they will poison your brain and your mind!

THE THOUGHTS THAT YOU THINK NOURISH YOUR MIND JUST LIKE THE FOOD YOU EAT NOURISHES YOUR BODY.

The body can convert food, but thoughts are trapped in your subconscious mind where they remain for the rest of your life.

If you are a mother, please help your children develop pleasing positive attitudes.

I can spot winners everytime, because of their enthusiasm and pleasing attitudes. When I meet their parents, without fail one or both parents has a pleasing positive attitude.

You actually poison your child if you are continually telling them "You're so sloppy," "You're so bad," or "You're no good."

By continually telling children these negative things you can literally destroy them.

Many parents destroy their children this way and they remain destroyed for the rest of their life.

They live with these attitudes about themselves.

Psychologists say the years from one to five are the most important years of development. However, all years are important.

An essential part of Super Fitness is a pleasing, positive attitude because it accentuates the positive, eliminates or solves the negative.

Your attitude is a key to being a SUPER WINNER and living a SUPER LIFE.

Be an upper, not a downer.

See the good in life and enjoy!

You can and will have a SUPER LIFE, but remember you have to earn it.

You have the potential.

Work hard to maintain a pleasing positive attitude — dream your dreams and make them come true.

Super Nourishing Environment

To continue developing a super pleasant attitude, it may be essential to change your negative destructive environments. That's right, change them.

If you are in a dark, dingy apartment and the dark dinginess makes you depressed, paint it yellow!

If you will notice, the colors of Super Fitness of America are yellow and orange and green.

They are happy colors.

They are living colors.

They are vibrant colors.

Get into an environment that's happy!

Whether you are working in an office or working in a dump, if the environment is bad, change it.

Get a new office.

Get a new job.

Destructive negative friends should be changed also.

If you have a negative boyfriend or girlfriend who is dragging you down the tubes continually, dump them!

If you have negative friends who are sucking the blood out of your spirit, abandon them!

I believe that loyalty is owed only to those who deserve it.

If you are loyal to someone who is destroying you, you can't help yourself or anyone else.

In order to help these people, you must have a pleasing positive attitude and any person or anything who destroys your attitude is not worth it.

They are destroying the quality of your life, your ability to help others, and your ability to enjoy life.

So remove yourself from negative environments — people and places.

Super Exciting Goals

Another way to gain a fantastic mental attitude is to set exciting goals clearly in your mind.

Have daily goals.

Have weekly goals.

Have monthly goals.

Have a goal in your life.

Why are you living?

Get an exciting goal.

One of my exciting goals is knowing I am going to help millions and millions of people.

I know how to help women trim their waist, hips and thighs.

I know how to firm arms and firm bustlines.

I know how to help their skin become more luxurious and vibrant.

I know how to make men and women have more energy and more enthusiasm.

I know how to make them think healthier thoughts.

No matter if they want to ski, swim, jump or just to be a mother or father or lover, I know that I can help them enjoy SUPER LIVING!

With men, I know how to trim their waistline which is their lifeline.

I know how to help them prevent heart attacks. According to the many published reports distributed by the National Heart Association, we know that people who are overweight, overfed and undernourished and mostly under exercised have more chances of becoming heart attack victims.

I know that chances of a heart attack are greatly multiplied if people are out of shape.

I know how to help children become healthier.

I know your children are what they eat and what they think and what they do.

So I know how to help your children build stronger bones and stronger muscles.

I know their teeth are dependent upon what they eat.

These are some of the exciting goals I have.

You have to put exciting goals into YOUR LIFE.

Setting goals and following through can be a very exciting way of life for you and your family.

Have an exciting goal, something you will work on every day.

SET YOUR SUPER EXCITING GOALS TODAY!

Break Out Of Your Rut

Another way to gain a pleasing attitude is to break out of your rut.

If you are doing the same thing every day, thinking the same thoughts, you are in a rut. Remember, the only difference between a rut and a grave is the depth.

You are digging that grave a little deeper each day until you end up in that grave and your life will be gone!

Get out of that rut, get some new clothes, have some new friends, meet some new people.

Get a new job or a hobby or go to a movie or do something new.

Get out of that same environment!

Environments can become stagnant.

Environments are either nourishing or toxic.

People are either nourishing or toxic.

Get into nourishing environments.

They help you grow.

GET OUT OF THAT RUT!

Develop some super new habits which will help you grow daily, such as reading new books, buying tickets to a series of concerts or taking a vacation every three months.

Look back upon your life.

What percentage of your life is left?

Live anew starting today the SUPER FITNESS WAY!

Keep Active

Another important ingredient of a super pleasing and positive attitude is to be ACTIVE.

Use your spirit each day.

Exercise your spirit.

The more you use your SPIRIT, the better it becomes.

The more you use your BODY, the better it becomes.

The more you use your MIND, the better it becomes.

So, keep active.

Physically active.

One of the basic laws of human physiology is: USE IT OR LOSE IT.

If you use your mind or your body, it gets better.

If it rests too much, it rusts!

People say, take it easy.

That's the problem, too many people are taking it easy.

Unfortunately, and I hate to say it, but the average person is more of a failure than a success.

They have more bills than bucks.

They are pressed down with the problems of the world.

They are worrying too much.

If you are vigorously using your mind and your body you are so strong and sharp you are not burdened with problems, because you SOLVE all problems that exist.

SO, KEEP ACTIVE.

USE IT or LOSE IT!

Count Your Assets

Another way to gain a super positive and pleasing attitude is count your assets.

Many people are complaining all the time about what they don't have.

As the saying goes, you complain about the quality of shoes you can afford until you meet the man who has no feet.

Your eyes are precious.

How much would you give for your eyes?

Would you give two million dollars for your eyes?

How about cutting off your arms?

What would you give for your arms?

How about cutting off your legs?

You do have priceless possessions so count your assets.

Control the Quality of Your Thoughts

Think pleasant thoughts.

Control your mind.

Your mind controls your destiny.

If you find yourself getting a negative attitude, CHANGE IT!

If you find yourself thinking something bad, think something good fast!

If you are around people who are making you feel bad, be polite and disappear!

I repeat. Control your mind and control your destiny.

Remember, the thoughts you are thinking are YOU!

As you think in your mind, so you become.

Control your mind, control your thoughts and develop a positive pleasing attitude.

I guarantee you, without a doubt, that if you will read this chapter every morning and every evening for thirty days and work on your attitude, your friends and family will notice the difference.

You will notice the difference.

You will be thankful to be alive.

You will make other people thankful they are alive.

You will bring happiness to others.

You will be better at your work.

Your boss will appreciate you more than ever.

You will be worth more.

Your whole life will change.

You have decided to think and act like a winner with a super pleasing positive mental attitude.

GET STARTED RIGHT NOW!!

Ten Commandments
of Positive Action for a Super
Pleasing Positive Attitude

1. Have love and faith in yourself.

2. See the good in all.

3. Regard problems as exciting opportunities and solve them.

4. Accentuate the positive, eliminate the negative.

5. Remove yourself from negative environments as soon as possible.

6. Keep exciting goals clearly in mind daily, monthly, yearly and lifelong.

7. Associate with pleasant positive people.

8. Break out of your rut and have the guts and determination to create the life you want.

9. Keep your mind and body active. BE A POSITIVE DOER.

10. Count your assets. ("I complained about no shoes, until I met a man who had no feet.")

Step Four

Part One
Super Exercise

Earn a Super Body by Super Exercise

You CAN earn a SUPER BODY!

The reason your body is so important isn't just for vanity's sake.

It is the temple of your spirit!

Without a strong vigorous body you cannot get through the struggles in life.

LIFE IS SURVIVAL OF THE FITTEST!

We're not talking about surviving in life but being triumphant in life!

Being triumphant over yourself!

Once you triumph over yourself, you can help others.

If you are not strong, you will not survive!

Many people literally KILL THEMSELVES.

I am convinced that most people commit suicide by thinking destructive thoughts, eating junk food, and by being physically inactive.

If you stop and think about it, you will realize that I am right.

People commit mental suicide because they are not inspired, educated or activated.

For a super body, you need physical activity known to all of us as exercise. It comes in many forms — swimming, jogging, or walking.

WALKING IS WONDERFUL. It's a natural movement and also a tranquilizer.

When you are walking you are relieving tension from your body and increasing circulation.

Your body actually circulates more blood by the contractions of muscles squeezing against your blood vessels than by the pumping action of your heart.

To help you earn a super body, I will help motivate you by telling you some of the benefits of exercise.

EXERCISE IS THE FOUNTAIN OF YOUTH!

Gloria Swanson is over 80 years old. She practices super nutrition, super thinking and super physical activities, and as a result, she looks fantastic.

How would you women like to be sexy and swinging at 80!

Let's face it, we are all human.

Getting lots of activity is not easy.

You have to be triumphant over yourself!

You have got to stop procrastinating and putting things off.

If I eat good food, it's not going to help YOUR body!

If I get activity, it's not going to help YOUR body.

It's what YOU DO that will benefit you!

So, the true battlefield which decides your triumph or your defeat in life IS WITHIN YOU!

You were born with potential.

YOU CAN DO IT!

All you have to do is realize you can win the battle over yourself.

Say to yourself, I am going to become master of my fate and captain of my spirit.

Now say, I AM MASTER OF MY FATE AND CAPTAIN OF MY SPIRIT!!

As you say this to yourself, you are giving yourself a positive thought.

YOU ARE BECOMING THAT WHICH YOU THINK!

Face the FAT!

Look in the mirror.

In order to have a super body, you have to face fat!

Look in the mirror, don't peek sideways or stand at your best angle.

Take your worst angle for a change and face the fat!

Look in your eyes and say, I will eat small portions of fresh natural foods slowly!

I believe that eating small portions of fresh natural food slowly is one of the many keys to successful weight loss.

Say to yourself, I will be physically active each and every day.

I will exercise my spirit vigorously.

I will win the battle of the bulge.

I will triumph over life.

You will be able to enjoy life if you are trim, firm, active and full of energy.

You will find yourself bouncing along through life.

Remember, you must keep physically active.

Use your body or you lose it!

The best single exercise for those of you who don't think you have the time to exercise is running in place.

Actually, you don't have the time NOT to exercise!

Run in place every morning before you take your shower. Stand on something soft such as carpet and run in place. Bring your knees up about one third of the way. Start by running in place for 15 seconds daily. Each day add five seconds a day.

Naturally, if you have heart or low back problems or other serious medical conditions check first with your physician.

By the time you are running for five minutes you will be in fantastic condition.

Your heart and blood vessels will receive a tremendous amount of exercise.

For women, running in place trims the waist, hips and thighs.

Your abdominal muscles, which are attached to your pelvis, keep you from falling over backwards.

Each time you run, you work the lower part of your waist.

Each time you pick up your thighs, it's working your hips and your rear. It's also working the muscles around your hips because these are attached to your thighs.

Running in place is really wonderful.

I suggest for people who want rapid results, run in

place in the morning and at night.

We are talking about a maximum of five minutes.

This exercise will tranquilize you.

It will increase your circulation.

It will actually pump blood up to your hair.

It will make your skin more luxurious.

It will help you remain youthful.

It will help you be sexy.

While we are on the subject of having a super body, I would like to mention super sex.

Be sure to read the chapter on SUPER SEX!

If you are running in place and keeping physically active, eating super food, thinking healthy thoughts and looking great, you will have more confidence.

When you have confidence in yourself, you can be creative.

You will become a super lover!

The other benefits of exercise are the tremendous stamina, strength and endurance you obtain.

Dr. Menninger, one of the founders of the Menninger Clinics, says, "Tranquilize with exercise."

I can't believe how many millions of people are taking tranquilizers.

I recommend you consider throwing away tranquilizers, uppers, downers, inners and the outers and stop eating junk food.

EARN SUPER FITNESS of your spirit, mind, body and attitude.

It's actually EASIER to live the SUPER FITNESS way of life.

Lots cheaper too!

As I stated, people are committing suicide.

I don't want this to happen to YOU.

You are MY student.

TRANQUILIZE WITH EXERCISE!!!

BE BORN ANEW!

Another key exercise to keep a trim and firm tummy is abdominal curls.

This is done by lying on your back with your feet flat on the floor. Put your hands behind your head, come up only one-third of the way. Breathe out as you come up and breathe in as you lower your upper body back to the floor.

Start with five repetitions, add one a day until you are doing thirty repetitions.

This will help trim and firm your waist.

It is tremendous for elimination.

Many people are constipated. By doing this exercise, it squeezes the abdominal muscles.

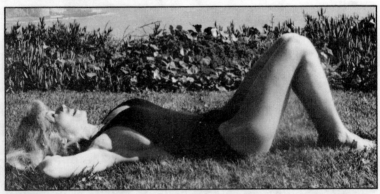

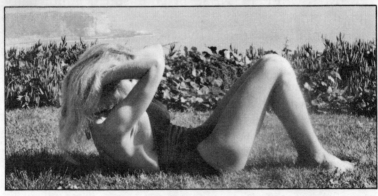

The third exercise is pushups.

Some people may wish to do "modified" pushups with knees on the ground.

Place your hands extended on the floor in front of you.

Breathe in as you go down, breathe out as you go up.

Start with five "modified" pushups and add one a day and do as many as you can. Do these three times a week. Monday, Wednesday, Friday, or Tuesday, Thursday or Saturday.

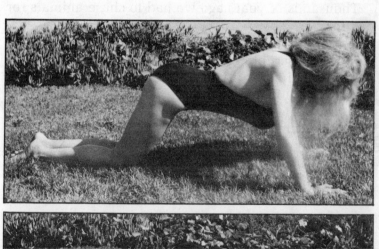

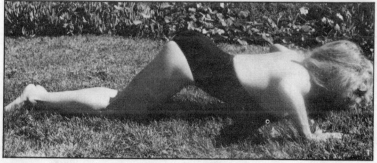

With the running in place, firming the hips, waist and thighs, the abdominal curls keeping your tummy firm, and the pushups, you're helping keep your whole supple body firm and strong.

You have no other choice!

It seems that the creator created life whereby we cannot be lazy.

People are looking for a gimmick! They are looking for an easy way to keep in shape.

You have to make physical activity as much fun as possible.

If you are lazy and overeat, you are going to grow old fast!

You will have a double chin, you'll get a pot belly, your tummy will sag, your thighs will be flabby.

You don't have any choice!

That's the way life was created!

Thousands of years ago we had to chase animals for our food.

We had to find or grow our own food. Women had to work hard, scrubbing clothes by hand.

Just existing required a tremendous amount of physical activity.

Now, we take a ride in a car, we have automatic machines, we are constantly looking for an easier way of life.

If you want to use these modern conveniences, you have to keep physically active.

Walking is wonderful!

Jogging is great!!

Be sure to wear shoes that protect you.

Run on a soft surface so that you don't hurt your back.

Swimming is sensational.

Tennis is terrific!

Hiking is fantastic!

The air that you breathe is one of the most important sources of nourishment for your body.

Next is the water you drink, followed by the food that you eat.

If you are living in a polluted area, move!

If you are drinking tap water, get bottled spring water!

And, naturally, eat fresh natural foods in their natural state.

Keep physically active and stay young.

The mind and the body and the spirit are one.

If your body is weak, you can't be spiritually strong.

If your attitude is lousy, it hurts your physical health. That's how people get ulcers, colitus, skin problems.

You are as strong as your weakest link.

Life is a struggle!

If you keep physically active, exercise regularly, eat fresh foods in their natural state, exercise your spirit and mind daily, you will be strong enough to solve the problems of life.

The goal that I want for you is to be SUPER FIT for a SUPER LIFE!

THAT IS YOUR NEW GOAL.

Exercise Is Super for Strength, Endurance and Flexibility

In order to develop super strength you have to do progressive resistive exercises.

The basic principle of these exercises is to do ten repetitions of the exercise until they become easy.

Then, add resistance.

By doing this, you can rapidly increase your strength.

During the first few months, many people can increase their strength by about 25 per cent.

With the strain of modern life, you need all the strength you can get!

Super strength is an integral part of SUPER FITNESS.

I was the United States National Bench Press Champion for six years.

My unofficial record was 350 pounds and officially, in contest, 320 pounds.

This experience has helped me to formulate my concept of SUPER FITNESS.

The other factor you need, of course, is endurance.

You EARN endurance by performing endurance activities.

If you are walking, walk faster and farther.

If you are running or jogging go a little farther each time.

If you are swimming, continually add a little more distance.

Strength and endurance are two of the components of super physical fitness.

Kenneth Cooper's book, *Aerobics*, provides an excellent guide on how to calculate the amount of endurance exercises you are performing.

Another component of fitness is flexibility.

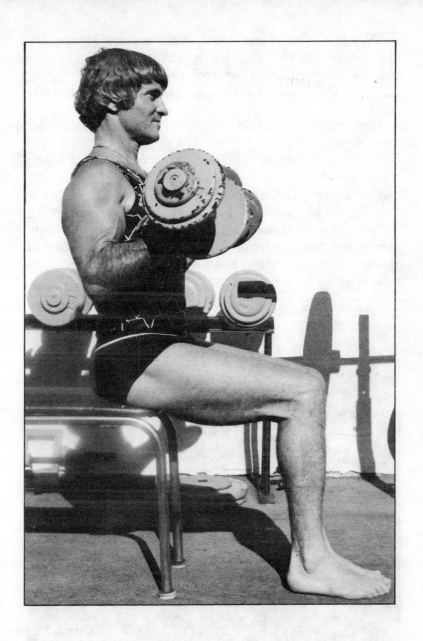

Two of the most commonly tight muscle groups are the hamstrings (the muscles in back of your thighs), and the low back muscles (erector spinal group).

To stretch your hamstrings, bend over, grab your ankles.

Holding your head down by your legs, straighten your legs slowly.

Now bend forward and straighten your legs and then bend again.

Do this five times and then relax.

Then do another set five times.

When you do this exercise you are holding your body down and you are using the front thigh muscles called the quadriceps to stretch out the muscles in the back of your legs.

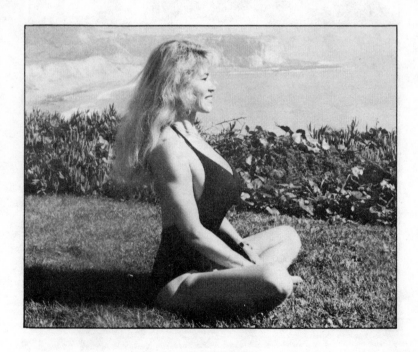

The other flexibility exercises that many people need is stretching the lower back muscles.

You do this by sitting on the floor and crossing your legs Indian style.

Now grab your ankles with both hands.

Breathe out and pull yourself slowly down, trying to touch your head to the floor.

Hold your head against the floor for five seconds.

For best results, repeat this exercise three sets of five repetitions each morning.

The other component needed for super fitness is skill.

Everyone should engage in some activity that requires coordination and skill such as tennis, golf, bowling.

Resolve this moment to engage regularly in physical activity every day, the rest of your life.

Regular physical activity will add years to your life and life to your years.

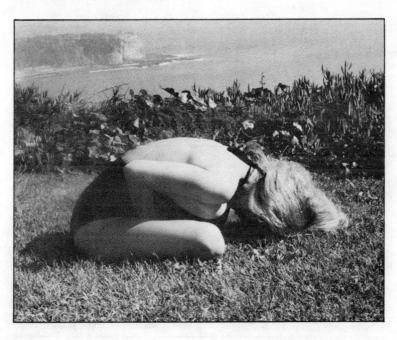

Physical Activity Caloric Expenditure Chart

Physical Activity		Calories per Hour
Walking	2 m.p.h.	200
	3 m.p.h.	270
	4 m.p.h.	350
Running		800-1000
Cycling	5 m.p.h.	250
	10 m.p.h.	450
	14 m.p.h.	700
Horseback riding		
	Walk	150
	Trot	500
	Gallop	600
Dancing		200-400

Physical Exercise	Calories per Hour
Gymnastics	200-500
Golf	300
Tennis	400-500
Soccer	550
Sculling	
50 strokes per min.	420
97 strokes per min.	670
Rowing (peak effort)	1200
Swimming, breast and	
backstroke	300-650
Crawl	700-900
Squash	600-700

	Calories per Hour
Climbing	700-900
Skiing	600-700
Skating (fast)	300-700
Wrestling	900-1000
Weight Training	500-600
Competitive Body Building	950-1100

Domestic Occupations	Calories per Hour
Sewing	10-30
Writing	20
Sitting at rest	15
Dressing and undressing	30-40
Ironing (with 5-lb. iron)	60
Dishwashing	60
Sweeping or dusting	80-130
Polishing	150-200

Industrial Occupations	Calories per Hour
Tailoring	80-130
Shoemaking	80-100
Bookbinding	75-100
Locksmith	150-200
House-painter	150-200
Carpenter	150-200
Joiner	200
Cartwright	200
Smith (light work)	250-300
Smith (heavy work)	300-400
Riveting	300
Coal mining (av. for shift)	200-400
Stonemason	300-400
Sawing wood	400-600

Dr. Jean Mayer, a super nutrition expert at Harvard, states that the effects of exercise on weight loss through increased calorie expenditure is cumulative — it adds up.

For instance, it would require seven hours of sawing wood to burn up 3500 calories — but you don't have to do it all in one stretch.

If you sawed wood for thirty minutes a day, it would add up to seven hours in two weeks.

If your calorie intake from food remained the same, you could lose twenty-six pounds in one year by spending a half-hour a day on the woodpile.

A half-hour every other day skating, tennis, swimming or a good workout at a health spa will result in sixteen pounds weight loss a year.

Some Benefits of Exercise

1. Improvement in your general appearance and the firming of flabby muscles.

2. Increased efficiency with less energy spent performing both physical and mental tasks.

3. Increased strength, endurance and coordination.

4. Improved ability to relax and to voluntarily reduce tension.

5. Reduction of chronic fatigue commonly due to lack of exercise.

6. Stimulation of blood circulation during exercise.

How to Trim Down
Your Waistline in 31 Days

Do the following for 31 days and the results will amaze you.

1. Take before and after photos of yourself, especially the side view and waist measurements.
   Let it all hang out!
   This will motivate you.

2. Practice SUPER DISCIPLINE for 31 days:
   a. Eat small portions, slowly.
   b. Fast on warm liquids, such as warm prune juice, one day a week. Make it the day when you are under the least amount of stress.
   c. For added nutrition insurance on this program, take your *Super Food Protein Drink* for breakfast and your *Super Packs* and *Staminal* regularly, as described in the section on food supplements.
   d. Do the sidebends and abdominal curls every morning and evening. Begin with a comfortable number of repetitions, say about fifteen, according to your age, physical condition, and add one repetition a day for 31 days.
   e. Tell yourself during the day:
   "My waist is getting trimmer."
   "I'm going to have the discipline to stick with this program."
   "I'm going to look SUPER!"
   "I'm going to feel SUPER!"
   "I'm going to have more energy!"
   "I'm going to be so proud of how I look in my new clothes."

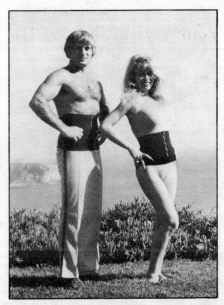

f. Wear a SUPER BELT.* It makes you more conscious of your waistline and helps you have that extra discipline. It also presses against your waist so psychologically you don't feel like eating as much food.

g. Tape a waist-measurement chart on your bathroom mirror and measure yourself daily. Set your goal of two or three inches at the end of the 31 days.

Of course, the size of your waist *the rest of your life* is the key.

But this 31-day waistline reduction program will help you get rolling.

To maintain that waistline just become waistline-conscious.

Never buy larger size clothes.

Follow the principles outlined in SUPER FITNESS and remember ... YOUR WAISTLINE IS YOUR LIFELINE!

---

* Super Belt™ — a Super Fitness of America product which binds the waist tightly.

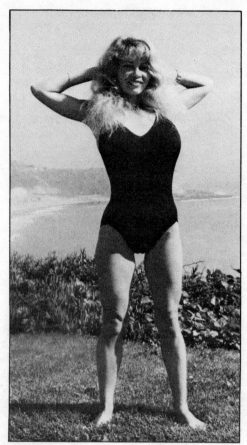

Fig. 1

Side Bends

Starting position: Feet apart, hands behind head (fig. 1). Bend to left with trunk forward at about 10 degree angle, knees slightly bent, and exhale (fig. 3). Breathe in and repeat same procedure to right (fig. 3).

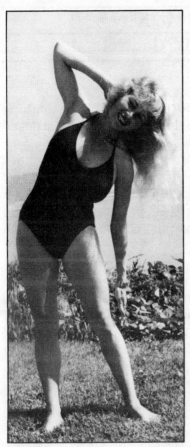

Fig. 2

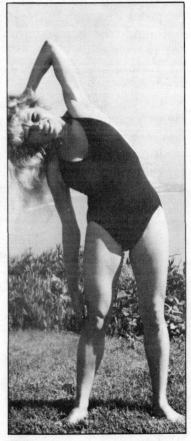

Fig.3

Physical Activity
For Weight Control

The fastest way to lose stored body fat is to combine increased physical activity (exercise) with decreased caloric intake.

Relating the caloric output of one activity to another is a tremendous aid in planning your SUPER new life.

You must know approximately how much energy you expend in order to determine how much and what to eat, and whether you are exercising too little, too much or improperly.

To lose one pound of fat a week, you would have to reduce your consumption of calories by 3,500.

Or you can use a combination of both approaches, which many doctors recommend, and is the one that I believe in.

Increase your physical activity and cut down on some of your meals, and you'll have no trouble taking it off.

The combination of increasing your physical activity and controlling the quality and quantity of your food intake is the key to controlling your bodyweight.

Remember the formula:

Decrease the quantity of food intake.
+
Increase the quality of food intake.
+
Increase physical exercise.
=
LOSE WEIGHT + FEEL GREAT.

Super Fitness Motivation

One of the keys to establishing and staying inspired to exercise plus keeping physically active is to keep a super accurate record of your progress.

I've created the following forms and charts in order to keep you enthused.

USE THEM!

Take your photos today in a bathing suit — front and side shots.

Then take your measurements.

Set realistic goals.

Fill in the body weight record.

Give yourself a daily score for your nutrition, exercise and attitude.

These records were created to help you achieve SUPER FITNESS.

Take the first step NOW!

Each step will help you feel better and look better. The more steps you take the more SUPER you will look and feel!

Fitness Photo History*

"BEFORE"

"AFTER"
3 MONTHS

FRONT Date: FRONT Date:

* Take photos as soon as possible after beginning fitness program in bathing suit.

SIDE Date: SIDE Date:

FACE THE FAT and see yourself improve!

Body Measurements

NOTES:

1. *Weight taken nude before breakfast, after bowel movement, same time each day.*

2. *Fitness educator must take your measurements to be sure they are taken accurately.*

	Starting Measurements	1 Month	2 Months	3 Months	GOALS
DATE					
Weight					
Neck					
Right Upper Arm					
Chest (Men) Bust (Women)					
Waist					
Hips					
Right Thigh					
Right Calf					

Weight Loss Graph

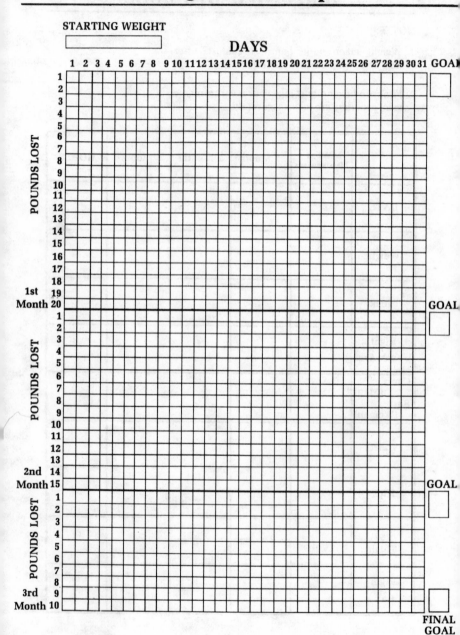

STARTING WEIGHT

DAYS

POUNDS LOST

1st Month

POUNDS LOST

2nd Month

POUNDS LOST

3rd Month

GOAL

GOAL

GOAL

FINAL GOAL

YEAR

82

Super Fitness Diary©

RATING SCALE

10 = SUPER!
8 = GOOD
6 = AVERAGE
4 = FAIR
2 = POOR
0 = BAD

	THOUGHTS AND ATTITUDE			NUTRITION			EXERCISE		
	1st Month	2nd Month	3rd Month	1st Month	2nd Month	3rd Month	1st Month	2nd Month	3rd Month
1									
2									
3									
4									
5									
6									
7									
8									
9									
10									
11									
12									
13									
14									
15									
16									
17									
18									
19									
20									
21									
22									
23									
24									
25									
26									
27									
28									
29									
30									
31									
Total Points									
Average									

Ten Commandments of Positive
Action for Super Exercise
and Physical Activity

1. Begin all exercises gradually.

2. Progress regularly in resistance for strength, and duration for endurance.

3. Exercise to music for motivation and enjoyment.

4. Vary exercise routine monthly.

5. Do not hold your breath while exercising.

6. Do at least a 15-minute exercise routine the first thing each morning after meditation.

7. Make exercise fun! Have an exercise partner when possible.

8. Take photos and measurements every three months — physical inventory time.

9. Engage in as wide a variety of physical activities as possible.

10. Walking is wonderful — for all ages. Walk as much as possible.

Step Four

Part Two
Super Nutrition

Overeating, America's Number One Nutritional Problem

I'm convinced that overeating, otherwise known as "stuffing yourself" with too much food, is one of the worst nutritional sins of the average middle-aged American!

Overeating overloads your digestive system.

If you overload your digestive system or your car or your washing machine or the electrical circuit of your house, they can't function as well!

Body systems as well as machines break down.

Symptoms of your digestive system having problems are burping, belching, constipation, diarrhea, upset stomach.

For these conditions, Americans consume millions of pills and spend millions of dollars.

When you overeat or overload your digestive system, you cause an excess strain on your various digestive organs.

Because many people swallow their food too fast, they don't allow the digestive juices in their mouths time enough to work.

Continual eating causes a continual flow of such juices. These overused digestive juices, such as hydrochloric acid and pepsin, force organs such as your pancreas, kidneys and liver to overwork.

Overeating also prevents proper assimilation of food because it clogs up the digestive tract with masses of bulk.

The faulty assimilation of food is, in my opinion, one of the major causes of poor nutrition.

It's not only what you eat, but what your body assimilates that's important.

Assimilation is one of the keys to SUPER NUTRITION.

By overloading your system, you interfere with proper food assimilation.

Many people are constantly constipated.

Their intestines are impacted and clogged with food and feces.

This is not a theory — it's a fact!

Not only does this interfere with the assimilation of nutrients, it also causes the abdominal wall to swell, adding to the size of your waistline and creating discomfort.

If that isn't bad enough, this clogging affects your blood stream and the nourishment that goes into every cell of your body.

This is frequently overlooked, yet it is an extremely serious problem.

No matter how much you may know about nutrition, chemical composition of food, chemistry of your body — physiology, anatomy, neurology, psychology — if you overload and super stuff your digestive system, you are literally committing slow suicide.

Overeating is one of the main causes of overweight and obesity.

Obesity is a disease that has infected over 50,000,000 Americans!

Overeating is one of the causes of a potbelly which is not just an accumulation of fat but also the visual results of impacted and distended intestines filled with decaying food and feces.

Overeating also causes the abdominal muscles to become overstretched.

Overeating literally wears out your digestive system.

I would like to plant a key phrase in your mind. This phrase, if observed daily, will help prevent overeating, overstuffing and over-clogging of your digestive system.

EAT SMALL PORTIONS SLOWLY! (S.P.S.)

The next tip is not to mix too many different foods together at the same meal.

Keep your combination of foods as simple as possible.

You will not only be more comfortable without that stuffed feeling, but you will look better because you will lose weight.

You'll feel great because you'll have more energy.

Your body requires a huge amount of energy to digest food. Overeating robs you of energy instead of giving you more energy, as commonly thought.

You'll have more stamina, more endurance, more sex appeal and you'll be better nourished.

REMEMBER — EAT SMALL PORTIONS OF NATURAL FRESH FOODS SLOWLY!

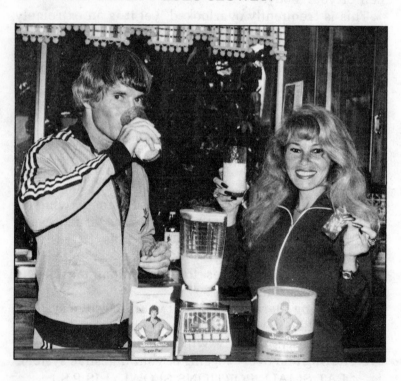

Fat is Fatal

The American Medical Association reports the following dangers from excess weight:

1. A 13% increase in death rates for individuals 10% overweight.

2. A 35% increase among those 20% overweight.

3. A 40% increase for those 30% over their normal weight.

Whenever an excessive deposit of fat accumulates on your body and your bodyweight exceeds its desired weight, you are becoming obese!

This condition may be slight (overweight) or gross (obese).

Most desirable weight standards are based upon height and weight tables put out by insurance companies.

Some of these weight tables are accurate and some are not.

The bony framework of your body as well as your height and weight must be taken into consideration to determine your optimum weight.

The following table was compiled by the U.S. Department of Agriculture.

It gives the approximate normal weight for the average man and woman.

Thirty percent of the obese reach the age of 70, while 50 per cent of the slim reach 70.

The age of 80 is reached by only 10% of the obese compared with 30% of the thin, a ratio of one to three.

Obesity encourages circulatory disorders, arthritis, gout, diabetes, heart disease and a host of other diseases.

Men			
Height	**Weight (without clothing)**		
without shoes	Light build	Medium build	Heavy build
5 ft. 3 in.	118	129	141
5 ft. 4 in.	122	133	145
5 ft. 5 in.	126	137	149
5 ft. 6 in.	130	142	155
5 ft. 7 in.	134	147	161
5 ft. 8 in.	139	151	166
5 ft. 9 in.	143	155	170
5 ft. 10 in.	147	159	174
5 ft. 11 in.	150	163	178
6 ft.	154	167	183
6 ft. 1 in.	158	171	188
6 ft. 2 in.	162	175	192
6 ft. 3 in.	165	178	195
Women			
5 ft.	100	109	118
5 ft. 1 in.	104	112	121
5 ft. 2 in.	107	115	125
5 ft. 3 in.	110	118	128
5 ft. 4 in.	113	122	132
5 ft. 5 in.	116	125	135
5 ft. 6 in.	120	129	139
5 ft. 7 in.	123	132	142
5 ft. 8 in.	126	136	146
5 ft. 9 in.	130	140	151
5 ft. 10 in.	133	144	156
5 ft. 11 in.	137	148	161
6 ft.	141	152	166

Medical researchers have estimated that your body must develop two miles of additional capillaries for every ten pounds of fat you accumulate.

This places an extra load on the heart and circulatory system that can prove fatal in the long run.

Heart disease and related circulatory problems claim over 500,000 lives annually in America!

FAT IS FATAL!

How To Diet and Lose Weight

CRASH DIETS ARE BAD!

The only crash diet I can safely recommend, if you want to call it that, is fasting on liquids plus food supplements one day a week.

If you'll keep physically active during that one day, nothing strenuous, you can lose up to two pounds in one day.

Food supplements are natural concentrated foods which assure your body that it's getting vitamins and minerals so necessary for its functioning.

You also need some bulk, such as bran.

This helps to cleanse your system and aids in your elimination.

You need a balance, that magic word "balance," with all your foods.

The ideal way to lose weight is to take the food supplements for added nutrition insurance and eat small portions slowly.

This really takes D-I-S-C-I-P-L-I-N-E because eating is so much fun!

Have some carbohydrates from fresh fruit but cut down on the quantity.

I recommend lean beef one or two times a week and also some fish, chicken and turkey which have fewer calories than beef.

Be sure to remove all the skin on fish and poultry before you eat it.

Don't cut out all your carbohydrates.

I don't believe in the no-carbohydrate-diet.

I do recommend the LOW carbohydrate diet.

I don't believe in any diet which does not contain all the essential food elements.

Carbohydrates provide energy; protein is needed to build your body tissues.

Fats are necessary for fuel and other vital functions.

Vitamins and minerals in your diet are essential to health and well being.

I believe in a delicious protein drink in the morning.

Many protein drinks will supply your body with 25 grams of protein, especially when made in a base of skim milk plus a fresh egg.

Papaya juice is also an excellent base for your protein drinks.

Cottage cheese is an excellent food.

Eat a nice green salad for roughage.

Mix all bran flakes in your foods or eat it straight with warm water or a soft boiled egg and warm water.

Soup is good on a diet because the warm liquid helps your digestion and elimination.

The main points to follow are:

1. Take natural potency food supplements.
2. Eat small portions slowly. (SPS)
3. Have a protein drink for breakfast.
4. Increase your physical activities.
5. Keep your intake of calories and carbohydrates down.
6. Stay away from unbalanced fad diets.
7. Stay away from junk foods.

In short, EAT LESS FOOD AND INCREASE your PHYSICAL ACTIVITY!

A good way to force yourself to have physical activity is to go to a health spa.

A big advantage of being at a spa is that you are away from the telephone, away from your children temporarily. This gives you a refreshing break and prevents interruptions and excuses for not exercising.

When you go to a spa, you go there for one thing, to exercise.

There are instructors there who will encourage and motivate you to exercise and lose those ugly pounds.

They have special equipment to help firm and tone your body.

Many have jogging tracks.

They usually have a warm therapy pool where you can enjoy relaxation and increase circulation in your body.

Remember, INCREASE your physical activity! Without cutting a single calorie, you can lose ten pounds a year by just walking a mile a day.

Researchers at Harvard have found that short periods of exercise do not make a person immediately hungry.

So, the idea that exercise only makes you want to eat more food is nonsense.

In fact, Harvard doctors found that lack of ACTIVITY always led to weight gain!

Take before and after photographs every three months, as directed in your personal Fitness Folder in this book.

When people look at themselves in the mirror, they see themselves from their best angle!

They don't face the fat.

You must face the fat!

When you see your photograph it is a tremendous motivator.

Take the photos, fill in your weight chart daily.

Set your GOAL for what you want to weigh at the end of each month.

Record the measurements in your Fitness Folder chart. This will help give you the discipline to control your mouth and what you eat!!

EAT LESS, INCREASE YOUR PHYSICAL ACTIVITY, and you HAVE GOT TO LOSE WEIGHT! Set the goal to develop SUPER DISCIPLINE and you WILL do it!

Party Reducing

Many of us can stay on our programs until someone calls and says, "Let's go to a party!" You want to go but may be afraid of spoiling your reducing program. Well, go ahead and go! But first, follow these simple rules:

1. Eat before going to the party — eat protein foods or drink half of a protein drink.

2. Take 12 Staminal one half hour before leaving.*

3. At a dinner party have a large portion of meat-fish-chicken or any protein, a large salad with vinegar and oil dressing.

4. At a cocktail party or going with a group to a cocktail lounge, eat only hors d'oeuvres that are protein, such as:
   meatballs or beef cubes
   scallops (no breading)
   cheese squares
   shrimp (no breading) or a shrimp cocktail
   carrot sticks, celery sticks, any fresh vegetable

5. If you must drink, have white wine or champagne.
   Most important, enjoy the party and the people. Don't make *food* the most important part of the party.

---

* Staminal — Concentrated tablets of natural B vitamins from liver and yeast.

Nutritional Program for Gaining Weight

The following nutritional program is designed for people interested in gaining weight. This program should be used in conjunction with an exercise program using maximum resistance done fewer times. Follow this program as long as you wish to continue to gain weight. Watch your waistline! Be sure the weight you are gaining is good solid weight in the right places.

1. Cut out all sugar and products containing sugar.

2. Eat three well rounded meals every day, using the following general rules.
    a. Have at least six ounces of any protein source at each of the three meals. Protein sources are: Fish, sea foods, poultry, eggs, milk, cheeses, meat.
    b. Have a minimum of two fruits daily.
    c. Have a minimum of one large raw salad daily.
    d. Have at least one cooked vegetable daily.
    e. Have no less than two but no more than four servings of any whole grain products.

3. Have as much of the following beverages as you wish — Milk, fruit and vegetable juices, water. Limit your intake of coffee and tea.

4. Take at least two Super Pacs daily.*

5. Have three Super Shakes (protein-based drink) daily, taking six Staminal tablets with each drink. The whole daily supply is shown on the next pages.

---

* Super Pac — Concentrated food tablets of Vitamins A, B, C, and D, lecithin, minerals — all derived from food sources rather synthetic sources wherever possible.

Supplement Protein Drink

Place in blender:	Calories	Protein Grams
1½ cups papaya juice	156	4
1½ cups whole milk	239	12
1 whole fruit	78	2
1 tbsp. honey	65	.1
2 tbsp. peanut butter (optional)	190	9
4 rounded tbsp. Super Food	200	51
Fill blender with ice	928	78.1
Divide into 3 equal parts	309	26

Drink 1 part 1½ hours after each meal.

Supplement Protein Drink

For lighter (under 150 lbs.)
or over 150 lbs. but inactive:

Place in blender:
    ½ Cup Papaya Juice
    ½ Cup Milk
Cover, start on low speed and add:
    2 Rounded tbsps
    Super Food
Turn off blender, add only one of following:
    ¼ Banana
    3 Strawberries
    ¼ Portion any fruit
Turn on high speed for 15 seconds. Add:
    1 Cup crushed ice or
    5 Ice cubes
Blend to desired consistency.

Place in blender:
    ½ Cup Papaya Juice
    ½ Cup Milk
Cover, start on low speed and add:
    2 Rounded tbsps
      Super Food
Turn off blender, add only one of following:
    ½ Banana
    6 Strawberries
    ½ Portion any fruit
Turn on high speed for 15 seconds. Add:
    1 Cup crushed ice or
    5 Ice cubes
Blend to desired consistency.

Drink entire mix for one meal. Take six Staminal tablets with each Super Shake Meal. The milk may be substituted with one teaspoon of pure safflower oil and one-half cup of water for people on low cholesterol diets or those not wishing to use milk.

The third meal is as follows:
1. Four to six ounces for lighter, less active; six to eight ounces for larger, more active, of any one of the following (or smaller portions of any combinations not to exceed total weight): Fish, sea food, chicken, turkey, cottage cheese, eggs, lean meat.

2. Large green salad with two to three tablespoons dressing made of safflower oil, cider vinegar and herbs (packaged dry dressing with no sugar).

3. Serving cooked, dark green vegetable.

4. One Super/Pak Snacks of any raw vegetable sticks are allowed. For occasional hunger pangs, a few cheese or leftover chicken or roast beef cubes may be combined. Drinks allowed are water, diet beverages, coffee or tea. (A small amount of milk may be used in the coffee or tea, but no sugar. Raw honey can be used sparingly.

Ten-Day Rapid Reducing Plan

This plan should be followed for a maximum of ten days. It must be followed for at least seven days to be effective. Follow the outline exactly, but remember that the success of any plan is completely dependent on sticking with it, and that requires motivation and encouragement.

This plan is for those following a regular program of exercise, especially the progressive-resistance type. It is based on improved and balanced nutrition, so it should suit almost anyone in good health. However, if you have any question about your relative health in conjunction with this plan, your doctor should be consulted. If you are ready, this is the plan that has proved successful for so many.

Replace two meals with a super shake as outlined. One should be breakfast, the other may be either lunch or supper. All meals should be at least three hours apart, but no more than four hours apart. No food should be eaten within three hours of the time you go to bed.

The best results will happen after three or four days on this program. Take a Super Pac with food or super shake — not with water only. You may lose inches far faster than pounds. Do not become discouraged — the weight loss will eventually happen. Exercise and natural nutrition are recommended for best results.

10 Day Rapid Reducing Diet

SUPER SHAKE

8 oz. Super Blend
2 heaping tablespoons Super Food
1 egg (optional)
3 strawberries (unsweetened) or ¼ piece of
banana — once a day — or ¼ cup cantaloupe

Blend Super Blend, egg, and fruit together 15 seconds. Add Super Food while blending, blend for 15 seconds more and add 1 cup ice (crushed). Blend until smooth.

DIET #1

BREAKFAST
1 Super Shake
Super Pac
6 Staminal Tablets

LUNCH
1 SUPER Pack (Take before 4 P.M.)
6 Staminal Tablets
Plus one of the following meals:

1. 4 oz. meat-broiled (fish, veal, beef, poultry-no skin, white meat, lamb)
¾ cup cooked vegetables (lightly) NO CORN, PEAS, BEANS, SALT, OIL, BUTTER, BREAD, MILK, OR ANY OTHER FRUITS!!!! (You may only have the above mentioned fruits and ONLY in your PROTEIN DRINK!)

Small dinner salad with 1-2 tablespoons low calorie dressing.

2. EATING OUT — Chef Salad with 2 tablespoons low calorie dressing.

3. Brown Bag or Lunch Bag — sliced turkey breast, chicken breast or beef, ½ cup low fat cottage cheese, small dinner salad with 1-2 tablespoons low calorie dressing.

DINNER —
1 Super Shake
6 Staminal Tablets

SNACKS — Celery sticks, cucumber sticks, 2 carrot sticks per day, ½ protein drink (no egg) only once a day as a snack.

10 Day Rapid Reducing Diet

BREAKFAST
1 Super Shake
1 Super Pac
6 Staminal Tablets

LUNCH
1 Super Pac (Take before 4 P.M.)
6 Staminal Tablets
Celery sticks, cucumber sticks, 2 carrot sticks
with 1-2 tablespoons low calorie dressing.
and
½ Super Shake (no egg)

DINNER
6 Staminal Tablets

1. 4 oz. meat-broiled (fish, veal, beef, poultry-no-skin—white meat, lamb)

   ¾ cup cooked vegetables (lightly) NO CORN, PEAS, BEANS, SALT, OIL, BUTTER, BREAD, MILK, OR ANY OTHER FRUITS!!!! (You may only have the above mentioned fruits and ONLY in your PROTEIN DRINK!)

   Small dinner salad with 1-2 tablespoons low calorie dressing.

2. EATING OUT — Chef Salad with 2 tablespoons low calorie dressing.

RECIPE FOR SUPER BLEND CONCENTRATE

In a quart jar
1 cup Super Blend
add
4 cups water
shake well.

This will make 1 quart and one cup of Super Blend juice. This quart of juice will make you four delicious super shakes. Keep in refrigerator.
Refrigerate concentrate after opening juice.

SPECIAL

SUNDAY BREAKFAST

"Strawberry Omelette"

3 egg plain omelette.

Fill with fresh crushed strawberries. Add a drop of diet sweetener and Fresh Whip Cream. Top with fresh whip cream.

One slice of whole grain toast.

Coffee or tea with cream.

One Super Pac/
Six Staminal

SPECIAL WEEKEND BREAKFAST
Drink

4 oz. whole milk
4 oz. of ONE of the following:
Pineapple
Apple
Orange
Blend.
Add:
2 tablespoons Super Food
¼ portion any fruit
3 ice cubes
1 tablespoon safflower oil
1 egg

One Super Pac/
Six Staminal

Questions On Dieting

1. Does eating before meals make for less total food intake?

   Yes. A low-calorie snack, such as Super Snacks, a protein drink, an orange, a carrot, or perhaps a salad, eaten 30 minutes before a meal will tend to make you eat less. The reason? In about half an hour the carbohydrate from the food has begun to enter the bloodstream and the brain's appetite controls have been appeased to some extent. (But do not use low-bulk, high fat, foods such as cocktail nuts in this role).

2. When you eat slowly, do you eat less?

   Yes. For the same reasons as above. Often the person gobbles food too quickly for the body to feel satisfied.

3. Is periodic starving a good way to lose weight?

   No. The scale readings go down at once partly because the digestive tract is emptied. But this does not signify an equivalent amount of fat loss. An unbalanced diet may result in fatigue and depression which may contribute to the dieter's return to old eating habits.

4. Can you lose weight while the scale readings stay the same?

   Yes. As the body loses fat and plump storage cells shrivel, water tends to fill out the tissue. The extra water you hold replaces the poundage lost, or may even exceed it. Often discouragingly, the first three weeks of reducing show no results on the scale. This phenomenon is one of the chief reasons why diets are abandoned. Be patient; stay with the diet. Suddenly the water will be released in extra urination, and there will be a sharp drop in weight.

5. Are dietetic foods lower in calories?

Not always. Remember, "dietetic" generally refers to low-sugar content, for persons such as diabetics. Calorie totals are something else. In one study, for example, regular chocolate cookies were found to have 82 calories per ounce, dietetic — 109. Similar findings were made among dietetic candies. Regular ice creams are hardly different in calorie content from the dietetic.

6. Should dieters go easy on salt?

Yes. Salt affects fluid retention in the body. Going easy on salt during the first phases of reducing can help minimize the discouraging appearance of no loss, which is due to extra water being retained.

7. Do cooking methods have some bearing on cutting calorie intake?

Yes. Obviously, boiling, baking and steaming are preferred to frying and sautéing. For people who want to watch calories, there is stick-proof cookware which eliminates the need to use butter, oil or shortening.

8. Can you reduce on meal-in-a-can liquid diets?

Yes. But doctors are unenthusiastic about the idea. Mainly, these diets provide about 900 calories a day which is awfully low for the large or active person. They are nutritively complete — except for calories, of course — but, like all "monotony" diets, they are hard to stay with and teach nothing about how to maintain weight level after the weight loss. They also lack bulk, which makes them intestinally undesirable for the long pull. In addition, they are usually made from synthetic ingredients.

9. Is taking alcohol in quantity occasionally a fast way to gain weight?
No. Alcohol does provide calories, which the body treats like any others. But when one consumes more than a little, some goes off as vapor from the lungs and some by rapid secretion into urine. From a caloric point of view, one is better off consuming several drinks at an occasional party than having a drink every day.

10. Most people gain weight when they stop smoking — is it better to go on smoking rather than get fat?
No. The typical weight-gain of a withdrawing smoker totals about seven pounds, an amount not really difficult to lose. On the other hand, it has been calculated that the bad physical effects of smoking may be akin to those carrying an extra 100 pounds.

11. Does grapefruit burn up fat?
No. There is no magical property to grapefruit.

12. How much water should a dieter drink?
As much as they want. The body maintains a perpetual balance "between the faucet and the bathroom."

13. What are weight plateaus?
Plateaus are periods in which there is no apparent weight loss. A common one is the Third Week Plateau, which involves a readjustment of the water balance in the system. If dieting continues, further weight loss will occur.

14. Why does a dieter lose more weight in the beginning of a diet program?
The first week often produces a larger weight loss because sudden dietary changes usually involves a decrease in salt intake, and therefore, an increased loss of water.

15. Does age or the amount of weight to be lost have a bearing on how quickly you will lose it?
Yes. The older you are or the less you have to lose, the slower your weight reduction will be.

Tips for a Faster Weight Loss

1. Never eat or drink unless you are truly hungry or thirsty.

2. Do not eat or drink on a coffee break just to be sociable unless it is unsweetened coffee, tea or preferably water.

3. Eat slowly. This gives the regulatory mechanisms of the body a chance to act on our appetite centers, reducing hunger during the meal and allowing us to be satisfied with less food.

4. Do not skip meals or it will be difficult to control your appetite when you do eat.

5. Never shop for food on an empty stomach.

6. Eat dinner early. This enables the body to burn up what it has consumed.

7. When you feel hungry, try having a liquid instead of eating. This may satisfy the urge for food.

8. Do not keep high calorie snacks around the house. Avoid temptation!

9. Keep low calorie snacks readily available — carrots, celery, fruits.

10. Eat a salad before the meal.

11. If you are going to eat late — eat less!

12. If you must have a sandwich — try to use only one slice of whole grain bread.

13. Do not fry meat; broiling, baking or boiling are preferable.

14. The best beverage is water.

15. Get plenty of rest. It is possible to mistake the body's need for rest for hunger pains.

16. Fish has more protein than beef and less calories.

17. No sugar.

18. Safflower margarine only.

19. Safflower mayonnaise only.

20. Safflower oil only.

21. No alcohol.

22. One ounce of cream or milk is allowed in each cup of coffee.

23. Herb tea — all you want.

24. No catsup.

25. Season with vegetable salt or spice.

26. Drink at least eight glasses of water a day.

27. Think trim!

28. Weigh daily.

29. Do not weigh one week before your period.

30. Do not weigh until your period is finished.

31. For those who must, white wine may be taken with dinner.

Problems Encountered During Reducing

1. *A weight gain.* It is a normal phenomenon for a person to see a gain of a few pounds. During weight reduction, water often accumulates, particularly in middle-aged and older women. This is simply because the fatty tissue and skin may not shrink back to the "pre-fatness" level as fast as the fat is being lost. The resulting empty space gets filled with water as the body tries to adjust to this loss. Water is HEAVIER than fat so it will show up on the scale as a gain. However, within a few days the skin and underlying tissues will shrink and the water will be lost.

2. *A plateau when no weight loss is seen although the dieter is dieting fervently.* This problem is also a result of the body adjusting to the weight loss. This is how it establishes its equilibrium at each new weight level. Also, through exercise, fatty tissue is being changed into healthy muscle tissue which is heavier than loose, flabby tissue — thus the plateau! Moreover, scientists have found that the longer the plateau — the greater the weight loss will follow.

3. *Skipping meals.* This is not a good way to reduce, and it usually results in over-eating. It is desirable to plan the diet around three or more meals a day, each meal containing adequate protein. When the daily food intake is divided into small portions and eaten at intervals, continued weight loss is more likely to occur.

4. *Crash dieters.* When the weight is lost too rapidly, the body doesn't have the ability to adjust to the new weight level — and the weight is usually gained back. There is also the risk of incurring serious illness. Some persons also experience weakness, dizziness, and the tendency to have anginal (heart) attacks.

5. *The menstrual cycle will have a definite affect on weight loss.* There is normally a weight gain from water retention. This should be taken into consideration when a weight loss program is started just before the period. It has even been noted that changing from poor eating habits to good eating habits, especially when taking food supplements, may speed up the cycle, bringing on the period and water retention earlier. Usually, there will be a gain in weight as much as four to ten pounds at the onset of the menstrual cycle.

6. *Sugar addiction.* "A little won't hurt?" For every ounce the body absorbs, 2.7 ounces of water is retained. Sugar acts as a catalyst, causing tremendous increases in weight way out of proportion to the amount of sugar consumed. Remember, all carbohydrate food, especially starches, pastas, flour products and desserts, are converted into sugar by the body.

FOOD SHEET

For this:		Substitute this:		
Beverages	Calories:		Calories:	Saved:
Prune juice	170	Tomato juice	50	120
Beer	175	Wine (dry)	75	100
Breakfast Foods				
Eggs (2 scrambled)	220	Eggs (2 boiled or poached)	160	60
Butter and Cheese				
Butter on toast	170	Applebutter on whole grain toast	90	80
Cheese (blue, American, swiss, etc.)	105	Cheese (cottage)	25	80
Desserts				
Angelfood cake 2″	110	Cantaloupe ½	40	70
Cheesecake	200	Watermelon	60	140
Pound cake	140	Plum 2	50	90
Apple Pie	345	Tangerine	40	305
Blueberry Pie	290	Blueberries 1 cup	45	245
Fish & Fowl				
Tuna (canned)	165	Crabmeat (canned)	80	85
Oysters (fried)	400	Oysters (fresh)	100	300
Fish sticks 5	200	Swordfish (broiled)	140	60
Lobster meat & butter	300	Lobster meat & lemon	95	205
Meat				
Loin roast	290	Pot roast	160	130
Hamburger (av. fat)	235	Hamburger (lean)	145	95
Porterhouse steak	250	Club steak	100	150
Rib lamb chop	300	Lamb, leg of	160	140
Pork chop	340	Veal chop	185	155
Pork roast	310	Veal roast	230	80
Pork sausage	405	Ham (boiled, lean)	200	205

For this:	Calories:	Substitute this:	Calories:	Saved:
Potatoes				
Fried	480	Baked	100	380
Mashed	245	Boiled	100	145
Salad				
Chef salad and oil	184	Chef salad & diet dressing	40	120
Chef salad and mayonnaise	125	Chef salad & diet dressing	40	85
Chef salad and creamy dressing	105	Chef salad & vinegar/lemon	30	75
Snacks				
Peanuts 1oz. salted	170	Apple	100	70
Soups				
Creamed (1 cup)	210	Chicken noodle	110	100
Bean	190	Beef noodle	110	80
Minestrone	105	Beef bouillon	10	95
Vegetables				
Baked beans 1 cup	320	Green beans	30	290
Lima beans	160	Asparagus	30	130
Corn	185	Cauliflower	30	155

Guide to The Selection of Foods for
Reducing Body Weight With High Nutrition

Unlimited Quantities With Moderation	Liberal Quantities	Limited Quantities
Fish	Cheese	Coffee
Sirloin Steak	Radishes	Tea
Lobster	Lettuce	Roquefort Cheese
Chuck Steak	Brussel Sprouts	Grapefruit
Crab	Tomato	Swiss Cheese
Pepper Steak	Cucumber	Nectarines
Sole	Green Beans	Bran Flakes
Round Steak	Wax Beans	Pickles
Flank Steak	Bean Sprouts	Melba Toast
Halibut	Spinach	Wheat Germ
Rib Steak	Alfalfa Sprouts	Vegetable Soup
Tuna	Beet greens	Safflower
Sardines	Mushrooms	Mayonnaise
Tenderloin Steak	Water Cress	Whole Milk
Hamburger	Bell Pepper	Croutons
Salmon	Rhubarb	Papaya
Eggs	Cantaloupe	Peach
Cottage Cheese	Endive	Egg Salad
Omelettes	Garlic	Carrots
Herb Tea	Vegetable Salt	Onion
Liver	Egg Plant	Tangerine
Prime Rib	Celery	Squash
Trout	Safflower Margarine	Apple
Turkey	Low Cal Dressing	Pears
Chicken	Safflower Oil	Avocado
Veal	Clear Soup	Cream
	Strawberries	Tomato Juice
	Asparagus	Caesar Salad
	Meat Loaf	
	Broccoli	
	Cabbage	
	Sesame Seeds	
	Cauliflower	

Very Limited Quantities	To Be Avoided
Corn	Alcohol
	Ice cream
Watermelon	Soft drinks
	Macaroni
Potatoes	Cocoa
	Red Beans
Oranges	Lima Beans
	Cereal
Bananas	Sweet potatoes
	Chocolate
Orange Juice	Raisins
	Figs
White Wine	Dates
	Crackers
Diet Drinks	Nuts (other than almonds)
	Sugar
Almonds	Pie
	Fruit cocktail
Grapefruit Juice	Cake
	Cookies
Pork	Cherries
	Syrups
Pineapple	Candy
	Pastry
Sunflower Seeds	Jelly
	Tacos
	Grape juice
Peanut Butter	Bran muffins
	Pretzels
Breaded Fish	Popcorn
	Gum
Ham	Rice
	Rolls
Corn Beef	Beer
	Salt
Raspberries	Garbanzo Beans
	Doughnut
Apple Juice	Jell-o
	Potato Salad or chips
Peas	Cream soups
	Cream cheese
Beets	Bagel
	Coconut
Honey	TV Dinners
	Hot Dogs
Apricot	Chili
	Pot pies

Super Habits to Trim Your Weight

FOOD	HOW MUCH TO OMIT	HOW OFTEN	LOSS PER YEAR
Butter or margarine	One pat	daily	5 pounds
Average layer cake	Half of one slice	weekly	1⅓ pounds
Breakfast ham	Half a serving	weekly	2½ pounds
Mashed potatoes	Half a serving	twice weekly	2 pounds
French fries	Half a serving	twice weekly	3 pounds
Medium fried bacon	two slices	weekly	3 pounds
Ice cream soda	one	weekly	5 pounds
Whipped cream	two tablespoons	weekly	1 pound
Mayonnaise	one tablespoon	weekly	1 pound
Baking powder biscuit (2½ in. diameter)	one	weekly	2½ pounds
Bread or toast	one slice	daily	6 pounds
Doughnut	one	weekly	2 pounds
Pie	half a slice	twice weekly	3½ pounds
Jam or jelly	one tablespoon	twice weekly	1½ pounds
Sugar	one teaspoon	daily	2 pounds
Rice	half a serving	weekly	1 pound
Canned fruit in syrup	half a serving	twice weekly	1½ pounds
Pork and beans	half a serving	weekly	2½ pounds
Beer	12 oz. can	weekly	2½ pounds
Carbonated drink	8 oz. glass	weekly	1 pound
Whiskey	1½ oz. glass	weekly	2 pounds
Wine	three oz.	weekly	1 pound
Most candies	one oz.	weekly	1½ pounds
Most cheese	one oz.	weekly	1½ pounds
Potato Chips	10 medium size	weekly	1½ pounds
Bread stuffing	half a serving	weekly	1½ pounds

Food Supplements, Natural
Concentrated Super Foods

I'm often asked the question: "Why should I take vitamins?"

I do not believe in taking vitamins per se.

I do believe in taking natural concentrated super foods which are rich sources of essential vitamins and minerals such as liver and yeast for the vital B vitamins; codliver oil for vitamin A and D; kelp for iodine and other minerals from the sea; vitamin E from wheat germ oil and minerals from bone meal; egg shells, dolomite and other natural sources. The Super-Pac contains these super-concentrated foods.

Artificial foods give you artificial nourishment. "Foodless Foods," foods containing mostly highly refined or artificial ingredients, are relatively lacking in essential nutrients. They constitute a huge percentage of the average diet.

In many cases people are OVER-FED and UNDER-NOURISHED.

They eat too much quantity and too few quality foods.

Their bodies are stuffed and starved at the same time.

Natural concentrated super foods and food supplements, supply large quantities of important vitamins and minerals in convenient easy-to-take tablets. These are added nutrition insurance.

I said, concentrated natural food tablets . . . not pills!

ALWAYS TAKE YOUR FOOD SUPPLEMENTS AFTER MEALS WITH LIQUIDS AND NEVER ON AN EMPTY STOMACH.

Remember, you BECOME what you EAT!

Natural, Synthetic and Crystalline Sources for Food Supplements

I recommend that you use food supplements from NATURAL sources. Read the label of the food supplements (commonly called vitamins) you are now taking and see if the source is
(1) NATURAL
(2) SYNTHETIC
(3) CRYSTALLINE

Item:	If source given is:	It Is:
Vitamin A	Fish Oils	Natural
Vitamin A	Acetate	Synthetic
Vitamin A	Palmitate-Lemon Grass	Synthetic
Vitamin A	Water Dispersible	Synthetic

VITAMIN B COMPLEX

Item:	If source given is:	It Is:
Vitamin B1	Yeast	Natural
Vitamin B1	Thiamine Mononitrate	Synthetic
Vitamin B1	Thiamine Hydrochloride	Synthetic
Vitamin B2	Yeast	Natural
Vitamin B2	Riboflavin	Synthetic
Vitamin B6	Yeast	Natural
Vitamin B6	Pyridoxine Hydrochloride	Synthetic
Vitamin B12	Yeast	Natural
Vitamin B12	Streptomycin fermentation	Crystalline
Vitamin B12	Cobalamin Concentrate	Crystalline
Para-amino-benzoic acid	Yeast	Natural
Para-amino-benzoic acid		Synthetic

Folic Acid	Yeast	Natural
Pantothenic Acid	Yeast	Natural
Pantothenic Acid	Calcium Pantothenate	Synthetic
Inositol	Soy Beans	Natural
Inositol	Reduced from corn	Crystalline
Choline	Soy Beans	Natural
Choline	Choline Bitartrate	Synthetic
Biotin	Liver	Natural
Biotin	d-biotin	Synthetic
Nicotinic Acid	Yeast	Natural
Nicotinic Acid	Niacin	Synthetic
Niacin	Yeast	Natural
Niacin	Niacinamide	Synthetic

VITAMIN C

Vitamin C	Citrus, Rose Hips, acerola berries	Natural (but fortified)
Vitamin C	Ascorbic Acid	Synthetic

VITAMIN D

Vitamin D	Fish Oil	Natural
Vitamin D	Irradiated Ergosterol	Synthetic
Vitamin D	Calciferol	Synthetic
Vitamin D	Activated Yeast	Synthetic

VITAMIN E COMPLEX

Vitamin E	Mixed Tocopherols	Natural
Vitamin E	Wheat germ oil	Natural
Vitamin E	d'Alpha Tocopherol	Natural
Vitamin E	d'lAlpha Tocopherol	Synthetic
Vitamin E	Water Dispersible	Crystalline
Vitamin K	Alfalfa	Natural
Vitamin K	Menadione	Synthetic

The Ten Most Commonly
Consumed Food Poisons

In my opinion, over 50% of all people are eating foods which literally poison their bodies every day.

Here are some of them, the top ten, that I would like you to STAY away from completely!

1. Refined Sugar.

I mean white, brown, green or purple! Sugar is found not just in the sugar bowl or in the sugar box, but hidden in cakes, pies, cookies, candies and the like.

Sugar is especially harmful because it deprives the body of critical nutrients needed to metabolize wholesome foods.

Sugar upsets the pancreas and floods the blood stream with glucose which robs the body of an adequate supply of this vital nutrient shortly after.

In my opinion sugar is responsible for speeding up the aging process as well as many other harmful effects.

2. Alcohol

I don't mean just hard liquor but also beer, wine and alcohol in other forms.

It's especially harmful to the body because it destroys brain cells in small quantities.

It upsets the function of the liver and destroys friendly bacteria in the intestines.

In short, it upsets the normal body functions and puts an excess strain on your liver and kidneys.

If you do drink I recommend white wine in MODERATION!

3. Tobacco.

Smoking interferes with the body's ability to obtain oxygen.

Your body needs oxygen in order to properly use any nutrient.

Kenneth H. Cooper, M.D., Author of *The New Aerobics*, says that smokers enjoy no conditioning effect from exercise while those who do not smoke enjoy a beneficial effect from exercising.

In other words, if you smoke and exercise, you'll get nothing from that exercise.

We all know smoking causes cancer! In a nutshell, smoking is suicide!!

4. Salt.

The ordinary table salt in iodized form you eat is harmful to your body.

It upsets the sodium potassium balance, constricts blood vessels, alters blood pressure in some people and leads the way to many internal diseases.

5. Nitrates and Nitrate Treated Foods.

Bacon, hot dogs, sandwich meats, smoked meats and all those similar products that look so good in your supermarket are bad for your health when they contain preservatives. Read the label.

I would rather you skip a meal than eat "junk meats."

6. Polluted Water.

There are nutritionists who believe that the inorganic minerals in water are important to your health.

The best source of minerals is your food.

Fruits, vegetables and food supplements are the very best forms.

The best form of water to drink for super health is bottled spring water.

7. Dirty air.

The condition of the air in our cities and surrounding suburbs has become a major concern to health officials — especially for those suffering from respiratory ailments.

However, it concerns all of us because oxygen is extremely important to the energy of the human body.

Contaminates in the air must be filtered out by the lungs and other body organs.

This is an unnecessary load on the body's purification system.

For many of us there is no way out of this daily contamination.

However, much of this bad air can be neutralized if you breathe in clear air 8 to 10 hours a day.

A friend of mine works in the heart of the City yet lives far out in the suburbs where he and his family get clean air.

It's a long trip for him every day, but he says it's proven beneficial to his entire respiratory system.

8. Aspirin and drugs in general.

A bottle of aspirin should have warning statements on its label.

People are unaware of the extremely dangerous effects of this little white pill.

For instance, when aspirin reaches the stomach it causes hemorrhaging in one form or another.

People take aspirin to kill pain.

However, pain is an important message from the body to the brain telling that somewhere in the body you are experiencing cellullar death.

It signals that somewhere in the body your very tissues are being destroyed.

Hiding such messages should not be your objective but rather the elimination of the cause of this destruction to your tissues.

I suggest you take aspirin only upon the direct advice of your physician.

9. Coffee and tea.

The caffeine in coffee and theophylline in tea destroy nerve cells.

In later years they play havoc with the memory.

Furthermore, blood sugar is lowered and this can have drastic effects on people with conditions relating to their blood sugar level.

10. Too much food!

Since I believe overeating is one of the major nutritional problems of the average middle-aged American, I have to include overeating in my top ten.

Overeating leads to obesity and fat kills!

Internal Cleanliness

Your body and digestive system must be given a rest from time to time from its job of food digestion and waste elimination.

A positive step is to rest the body for a 24-hour period from all foods.

In other words, by fasting.

I would like you to fast once a week on fresh juice!

Carrot and parsley or diluted grape juice is excellent.

You can drink all the juice you want and also take balanced natural food supplements, such as the SUPER-PAC.

In fact, you'll start looking forward to the "fast" day because of the light clean sensation you'll be giving your body.

This kind of tissue cleansing is not as popular in the United States as it is in other countries.

It is important to remember that fasting permits the body to keep itself "clean" and strengthens it.

Keep in mind that even though help against bacterias may come from drugs and medicines, they do not heal the body.

The body must heal itself.

Most drugs and medicines only help the body to live with the disease until its own immune functions and restorative processes can return the body to health.

Sickness is often a sign of a health crisis in the body. The body is demanding a rest from all food and a chance to cleanse itself.

These crises are harmful and accelerate the aging process.

It is much better to offer the body a planned rest from food than to have it become sick and demand a forced rest.

Smoking Is Suicide

Now let's have a little discussion about smoking.

This section is derived mostly from research.

I decided to use this information, even though it is not original, because I want to help you to stop smoking.

In my opinion, smoking is suicide!

If you have a death wish, if you are self-destructive, if you want to have bad breath, yellow fingers, congested lungs, turn off beauties of the opposite sex and waste money, then smoke!

The Handbook of Poisons, a classic among medical books, states that nicotine first stimulates, then depresses and paralyzes the cells of the peripheral autonomic nervous system. The autonomic nervous system controls the regulatory mechanism of the body — our most important defense mechanism. Dr. Alexander Berglas points out that a failure of the body defense mechanism is one of the predisposing factors in cancer.

It has been proven that smoking causes cancer of the throat and the lungs. Dr. Berglas further mentions why the use of tobacco is responsible for lung cancer. He points out that "Smokers may be more susceptible to lung cancer because their mucus membranes are often chronically inflamed. Smog irritates the bronchial tubes. Smog-plus-tobacco-plus-smoke result in a greater susceptibility."

You want cancer?

Then smoke!

Nicotine is a nerve irritant, not a relaxant as many people think. If you are smoking to calm your nerves, you are, in reality, stimulating and irritating them.

Eyesight can be impaired by too much smoking, not only from the smoke itself, but from the nicotine that erodes the nerve endings of the eye. Tobacco amblyopia (a gradual loss of vision) is an eye disease that can only be cured by giving up smoking.

When you breath air that is heavy with smoke — whether it is your cigarette or that of some inconsiderate person — the cells in your body tissues are weakened from lack of oxygen. Doctors call this *hypoxia*.

Heart disease is, without a doubt, greatly aggravated by smoking. Some doctors even think smoking causes heart diseases. The mortality rate from heart disease is 82% greater among smokers than non-smokers. Those who smoke more than one pack a day have a death rate of 95% greater than the non-smoker!

Putting It All Together

In a few short pages, you've been introduced to many topics about which hundreds of books have been written.

I want to expose you to a very broad area of study in hope you will continue to study on your own in your search for SUPER FITNESS.

Set special goals for yourself right now and make nutrition education an adventure.

Apply the knowledge to your daily living.

Change your food habits and you'll change your life for the best.

Do not fear the loss of a favorite food but rather look forward to new experiences with new SUPER FOODS!

REMEMBER, IF YOU EAT JUNK YOU WILL BECOME JUNKY!

High Protein and No Carbohydrate Foods

Meat	Portion	Calories	Protein Grams	Carbo-hydrates Grams
Steak — lean				
Round	Avg.	226	23	0
Swiss	Avg.	210	34	0
Tenderloin	4 oz.	225	34	0
Filet Mignon	Avg.	250	15	0
Sirloin	3 oz.	330	20	0
Chuck	Avg.	250	40	0
Roast Beef (lean)	4 oz.	206	33	0
Pot Roast	3 oz.	245	23	0
Heart (baked)	4 oz.	214	36	0
Hamburger (lean)	3 oz.	185	23	0
Hamburger (reg.)	3 oz.	245	21	0
Boiling Beef	3 oz.	245	23	0
Corned Beef	4 oz.	245	30	0
Dried Beef	4 oz.	230	38	0

Fish and Seafood	Portion	Calories	Protein Grams	Carbo-hydrates Grams
Pike	4 oz.	90	20	0
Filet of Sole	4 oz.	85	19	0
Codfish	4 oz.	180	32	0
Herring	4 oz.	200	19	0
Sea Bass	4 oz.	105	22	0
White Fish Baked	4 oz.	210	17	0
Red Snapper	4 oz.	100	22	0
Pompano Broiled	4 oz.	185	20	0
Perch Broiled	4 oz.	130	22	0
Haddock Broiled	4 oz.	135	20	0
Halibut Broiled	4 oz.	200	29	0
Flounder Broiled	4 oz.	70	17	0
Swordfish Broiled	4 oz.	200	32	0
Tuna, canned in oil	4 oz.	227	32	0

Salmon, canned pink	4 oz.	160	23	0
Mackerel, canned	4 oz.	205	24	0
Sardines, canned in oil	4 oz.	233	27	0
Lox, smoked	4 oz.	240	20	0

Poultry and Eggs	Portion	Calories	Protein Grams	Carbo-hydrates Grams
Chicken — Broiled	4 oz.	155	27	0
Chicken — Canned/ boned	4 oz.	226	24	0
Chicken — Barbecued	4 oz.	210	27	0
Chicken — Roasted	4 oz.	285	30	0
Capon — Roasted	4 oz.	320	24	0
Duck — Roasted	4 oz.	190	22	0
Turkey — Roasted	4 oz.	250	36	0
Eggs — Boiled	2	160	12	trace
Eggs — Poached	2	160	12	trace
(plain) Omelet	2	160	12	trace

Lamb	Portion	Calories	Protein Grams	Carbo-hydrates Grams
Lamb Chop Broiled	1 med/4 oz.	385	26	0
Lamb Patty	4 oz.	225	31	0
Lamb Roast/leg	4 oz.	320	30	0
Lamb Roast	4 oz.	390	25	0

Pork	Portion	Calories	Protein Grams	Carbo-hydrates Grams
Ham, Baked	4 oz.	320	19	0
Ham, Boiled	4 oz.	300	20	0
Ham, Steak	Avg. svg.	230	33	0
Pork Chop Broiled/baked	1 med	275	30	0
Pork Loin Roast	Avg. svg.	405	27	0
Pork Loin Chop/ center-cut	4 oz.	380	24	0

Protein Foods with Limited Carbohydrates

Meat and Meat Dishes	Portion	Calories	Protein Grams	Carbo-hydrates Grams
Bacon, 2 strips, crisp		100	5	1
Bacon, Canadian, broiled	2 oz.	155	16	trace
Beef Liver, broiled	4 oz.	260	30	6
Beef Stew	4 oz.	105	7.5	7.5
Bologna (4½″ slice)	4 slices	345	14	1
Corned Beef Hash	3 oz.	155	7	9
1 Frankfurter — 1 Cup Sauerkraut	1 svg.	200	8	10
Knockwurst	4 oz.	310	16	trace
Meat Balls	4 oz.	230	18	4
Meat Loaf	4 oz.	225	17	3
Polish Sausage	4 oz.	340	18	1

Vegetables	Serving	Calories	Protein Grams	Carbo-hydrates Grams
Asparagus	½ Cup	18	2	3
Tomato, fresh	1 med.	35	2	7
Tomato, stewed	8 oz.	50	2	10
Tomato, juice	8 oz.	45	2	10
Turnips, cooked	1 Cup	35	1	8
Beets, diced	½ Cup	25	1	6
Bermuda Onion, raw	4 oz.	50	2	10
Broccoli, cooked	1 Cup	40	5	7
Brussels Sprouts	1 Cup	45	5	8
Cabbage, Steamed	1 Cup	35	2	7
Carrots, canned	1 Cup	45	1	10
Carrots, 5½″ Raw	2 Carrots	40	2	10
Cucumber, 7½″ x 2″	1 Raw	30	1	7
Cauliflower, cooked	1 Cup	25	3	5

Celery, fresh				
8" x 1½"	1 Stalk	5	trace	2
Green Beans, fresh	1 Cup	30	2	7
Green Peppers, fresh	1 Med.	15	1	3
Spinach	1 Cup	40	5	3
Squash, Summer	1 Cup	30	2	7
Squash, Zucchini	8 oz.	40	2	8
Lettuce, 4¾"	¼ Head	15	1	3
Mushrooms, canned	½ Cup	20	2½	3
Onions, cooked	½ Cup	30	1.5	7
Onion, Raw				
Bermuda	1-2½"	40	2	10
Onions, Young Green	12-Topless	40	2	10
Parsley	4 Tb.	4	trace	trace
Peas	½ Cup	68	4½	10
Sauerkraut, canned	1 Cup	45	2	9

Poultry Dishes	Serving	Calories	Protein Grams	Carbo-hydrates Grams
Fried Chicken	½ Breast	155	25	1
Chicken Ala King	4 oz.	215	14	4
Chicken Aspic	4 oz.	30	2	2
Chopped Chicken Livers	2 oz.	285	6	5
Chicken Salad	4 oz.	230	28	4
Chicken Chop Suey	4 oz.	140	11	7
Creamed Chicken	4 oz.	400	35	8
Chicken Egg Foo Yung	1 svg.	185	20	4
Chicken Chow Mein	4 oz.	115	16	6

Nuts (roasted-salted)	Serving	Calories	Protein Grams	Carbo-hydrates Grams
Almonds	¼ Cup	212	6	7
Brazil	¼ Cup	239	5	4
Peanuts	¼ Cup	210	9	7
Pecans	¼ Cup	185	2.5	4
Cashew	¼ Cup	190	6	10

Seafood	Serving	Calories	Protein Grams	Carbo-hydrates Grams
Abalone, broiled	4 oz.	100	21	3
Clams, steamed	5 oz.	107	18	4
Lobster Tails	4 oz.	100	18	1
Fish Sticks	5 sticks/4 oz.	200	19	7½
Cherrystone Clams	6 Clams	100	15	5
Lobster — Broiled	½ avg.	125	18	trace
Crabmeat, canned	3 oz.	85	15	trace
Perch, Breaded	4 oz.	260	21	8
Clam Chowder, Manhattan	6 oz. Bowl	45	2	6
Oyster Cocktail	10 raw med.	80	10	4
Shrimp, canned	4 oz.	125	26	2
Scallops, Broiled	1 svg.	140	27	2

Dairy Foods	Serving	Calories	Protein Grams	Carbo-hydrates Grams
Cheese, American	1 oz.	70	4	trace
Cheese, Bleu	1 oz.	105	6	1
Cream Cheese, Spread	1 oz.	105	2	1
Cheese, Velveeta	1 oz.	105	7	1
Cheese, Roquefort	1 oz.	105	6	1
2 Egg Omelet with 1 oz. Cheese		260	18	1
Cottage Cheese-low fat	1 Cup	195	38	6
Cottage Cheese-creamed	1 Cup	195	38	6
Butter	1 Tb.	100	trace	trace
Half & Half Cream	4 oz.	163	4	5½
Whole Milk	4 oz.	80	4.5	6
Nonfat Milk	4 oz.	45	4.5	6½
Yogurt	½ Cup	60	4	6½

Fruits	Serving	Calories	Protein Grams	Carbo-hydrates Grams
Strawberries, fresh	¾ Cup	42	trace	10
Avocado, fresh	½ or 5 oz.	185	2	6
Cantaloupe	½ avg.	30	1	7
Lemon juice	1 Tb.	5	trace	1
Canned Peaches — water pk.	½ Cup	38	trace	10
Canned Pears — water pk.	½ Cup	40	trace	10
Plums, fresh	1 only	25	trace	7
Apple	½ (2½″)	35	trace	9
Cherries, fresh	½ Cup	40	1	10
Grapefruit, fresh sections	½ Cup	40	trace	10
Orange, fresh	½	30	1	8

Canned ready to serve with water added.

Soups	Serving	Calories	Protein Grams	Carbo-hydrates Grams
Chicken Noodle	1 Cup	65	4	8
French Onion	1 Cup	120	10	10
Chicken Gumbo	1 Cup	60	4	7
Minestrone	¾ Cup	80	4	10
Beef Noodle	1 Cup	70	4	7
Beef Bouillon	1 Cup	30	5	3

Foods High in Carbohydrates

Breads and Pastries	Serving	Calories	Protein Grams	Carbo-hydrates Grams
White bread	1 slice	60	2	12
Corn Muffin	1 only	150	3	23
French bread	1 slice (avg.)	60	2	12
Whole Wheat Bread	1 slice	60	2	12
Raisin Bread	1 slice	60	2	12
Rye Bread	1 slice	55	2	12
Pumpernickel Bread	1 slice	60	5	12
Date Nut Bread	1 slice	100	1	21
Banana Bread	1 slice	120	4	22
Apple Pie	Avg. svg.	345	3	51
Cherry Pie	Avg. svg.	355	4	52
Custard Pie	Avg. svg.	280	8	30
Cream Pie	Avg. svg.	480	20	55
Pumpkin Pie	Avg. svg.	275	5	66
Almond Macaroon	1	100	1	16
Cup Cake	1 Avg.	185	2	30
Chocolate Layer Cake Iced	Avg. svg. (2″)	445	5	67
Angel Food Cake (2″)	1 slice	110	3	24
Coffee Cake with nuts	1 piece	240	4	33
Fruit Cobbler	1 sml. svg.	200	1	44
Doughnut, jellied	1	245	3	37
Whole Wheat Muffins	1 Avg.	115	2	19
Pancakes, griddle	1-5″	75	3	11
French Toast — syrup	1 slice	150	4	23
Waffle, plain	1 med.	210	7	28
Rye Wafers	4	90	4	20
Soda Crackers	4	100	2	16
Corn Flakes	1 oz.	110	2	24

Shredded Wheat	1 Biscuit	100	3	23
Wheat Germ	1 Cup	245	18	32
Cooked Oatmeal	1 Cup	130	5	23
Rice	1 Cup	185	3	41
Cream of Wheat	1 Cup	100	3	21
Cooked Cereal	4 oz.	70	2	14
Dry Cereal (avg.)	4 oz.	100	2	15
Raisin Bran	1 Cup	80	2.5	17
Bran Cereal	½ Cup	60	2	16

Dairy Foods and Desserts	Serving	Calories	Protein Grams	Carbo-hydrates Grams
Milk, whole	8 oz.	160	9	12
Milk, Chocolate — Non fat Milk	8 oz.	190	8	27
Milk, Nonfat	8 oz.	90	9	13
Milk, Buttermilk	8 oz.	90	9	13
Ice Cream, Chocolate	1 scoop	150	3	14
Ice Cream, Vanilla	1 scoop	150	3	14
Chocolate Malt	8 oz.	280	13	32
Chocolate Sundae	Avg.	320	7	54
Ice Milk	1 Cup	285	9	42
Custard	1 Cup	285	13	28
Carmel Pudding	4 oz.	170	3	29
Tapioca Pudding	4 oz.	175	6	24
Gelatin Dessert ready-to-eat-plain	1 Cup	140	4	34
Sherbet, Orange	1 Cup	260	2	59
Yogurt (plain)	8 oz.	120	8	13

One Course Meals	Serving	Calories	Protein Grams	Carbo-hydrates Grams
Beef Pot Pie	Avg.	560	23	43
Chicken Pot Pie	Avg.	535	23	42
Macaroni & Cheese	1 Cup	470	18	43
Spaghetti & Meat Balls	1 Cup	335	19	39
Beef Stew & Vegetables	1 Cup	210	15	15
Pizza, Cheese	5½" piece	185	7	27
Spaghetti — Tomato & Cheese Sauce	1 Cup	260	9	37
Stuffed Bell Pepper	1 Avg.	155	14	11

Vegetables	Serving	Calories	Protein Grams	Carbo-hydrates Grams
Beans, baked	4 oz.	135	8	24
Butter Beans	4 oz.	125	6	23
Corn, fresh, frozen	4 oz.	115	4	23
Corn on Cob, 1 small		100	3	20
Kidney Beans	1 Cup	112	7	21
Peas, green	4 oz.	80	6	14
Potatoes, hash brown	4 oz.	260	3	33
Potato, baked	4 oz.	125	4	28
Potato, boiled	4 oz.	75	2	15
Potato, mashed	½ Cup	75	2	15
Potato, french fried	6 pieces	100	1	12
Sweet Potatoes, canned	1 Cup	285	5	54
Sweet Potatoes, baked	5 oz.	200	3	45

Fruits and Fruit Juices	Serving	Calories	Protein Grams	Carbo-hydrates Grams
Apple — fresh	1 (2½″)	70	trace	18
Apple — baked	1 lg./sugar	200	trace	50
Apple — sauce/ fresh/unsweetened	4 oz.	50	trace	13
Banana 6″ x 1½″	1 med.	85	1	23
Blackberries — fresh	1 Cup	85	2	21
Blueberries — fresh	1 Cup	85	1	21
Cherries, sweet — fresh	1 Cup	80	2	20
Dates, pitted	1 Cup	490	4	130
Pineapple — fresh	1 Cup	75	1	19
Fruit Cocktail, canned	1 Cup	195	1	50
Grapefruit	½ Avg.	55	1	14
Orange — fresh	1 med.	60	2	16
Apple juice	4 oz.	60	trace	15
Cranberry juice	8 oz.	160	trace	41
Orange juice — fresh	8 oz.	115	2	26
Grapefruit Juice — unsweetened	8 oz.	100	1	24
Pineapple juice	8 oz.	135	1	34
Grape juice	8 oz.	165	1	42
Prune juice	8 oz.	200	1	49
Watermelon, fresh 4″ x 8″	1 Wedge	115	2	27

Beverages	Serving	Calories	Protein Grams	Carbo-hydrates Grams
Coffee — black	8 oz.	0	0	0
with cream/sugar	8 oz.	50	trace	5
with skim milk	8 oz.	5	trace	trace
with non dairy creamer	8 oz.	11	trace	1.0
Beer	12 oz.	125	trace	13
Highball	8 oz.	70	trace	18
Wine cooler	8 oz.	150	8	11
Sherry	1 glass	115	trace	5
Carbonated Seltzer water	8 oz.	0	0	0
Burgundy	1 glass	75	trace	4
Cola — reg.	8 oz.	109	0	27
Cola — diet	8 oz.	2	0	0
Orange Soda	8 oz.	110	0	28
Tea — plain	8 oz.	0	0	0

Jam, Jelly & Sweets	Serving	Calories	Protein Grams	Carbo-hydrates Grams
Apricot Jam	1 Tbsp.	50	trace	14
Grape Jam	1 Tbsp.	55	trace	14
Most Jams	1 Tbsp.	55	trace	14
Most Jellies	1 Tbsp.	55	trace	13
Honey	1 Tbsp.	65	trace	17

Ten Commandments of Positive Action for Super Nutrition

(1) Eat small portions slowly. (S.P.S.)

(2) Eat fresh food as close to the natural state as possible.

(3) Refrain from sugar, preservatives, pesticides, artificial additives, steroids, salt and fried foods.

(4) Rest the digestive system one day a week on freshly squeezed fruit juices and natural potency food supplements.

(5) Take natural concentrated super foods (food supplements) after each meal.

(6) Eat in a pleasing relaxed atmosphere.

(7) Eat foods created by nature, not artificially created by man.

(8) Chew food thoroughly to promote assimilation and prevent constipation.

(9) Drink natural liquids from natural sources and spring water.

(10) PRACTICE SUPER NUTRITION.

The Pay Off — Super Living
Super Sex

SUPER FITNESS LEADS TO SUPER SEX!

Please understand when I say SUPER SEX I am not saying that it is in any way evil, dirty or naughty.

My attitude toward sex is that it is one of the most natural things we humans engage in!

Without sex, the human race would end!

For the billion or more people on earth, sex is one of the few luxuries that they have to enjoy!

I don't need to justify sex, I only want to say that when you are in super shape, you can enjoy super sex.

The reason is, WHEN YOU LOOK SUPER, you can "turn on" your mate!

You're going to get him or her excited!

You are going to look so good that they are going to be interested, stimulated and whatever other words you want to use!

They are going to be turned on naturally.

If you are a woman you are not going to have to worry about wearing artificial breasts, artificial hair or an artificial rear end!

You are going to turn people on naturally because you look super!

If you're a man, you're going to have a trim waist, you're going to have a strong virile body bursting with energy and when these two super people who look great and feel great, have boundless energy, stamina and endurance get together, that's what I mean by SUPER SEX!

It's clean as a whistle.

It's natural and it's SUPER!

Did you ever stop to think that sex is an emotional and mental activity as well as a physical activity?

You have to be in shape mentally as well as physically.

You have to be sure of yourself.

You have to know that you have what it takes!

You get this super confidence from controlling your mind.

From knowing that you have the super body, mind and mental attitude to leave your partner in ecstacy!

Confidence comes from knowing you are in super shape.

You feel so secure and so confident that you are bursting with energy and vitality.

You have to have confidence to be a creative lover.

You don't have to read a book on the one-two-three steps of sex or the five easy steps to become a great lover.

Your confidence will come from inside you, not from outside sources such as books and lectures.

You will not be afraid of trying new sexual adventures.

Most people who have been lovers for years are doing the same old love routine all the time.

It can get pretty stale.

So you have to be creative.

People have confided to me that they've made love to the same person for over ten years and every time it's been different, because they are super fit mentally and physically, super confident and thus, super creative.

I'm talking about mental fitness, the confidence that allows you to be creative and I'm repeating it because when you have confidence in yourself and your capabilities, and your mind is positive and pleasing, you have a pleasing positive personality. With this strength and energy and endurance and stamina, you're a winner!

Being super at sex is no different than being super at a profession, such as being a super cook or a super artist or whatever.

Practice makes perfect!

And I don't mean that as a joke.

There are no limits to the sexual creativity that lies dormant within you.

If you are sexually creative, your mate will hang onto you for dear life for the rest of your life!

They'll never let you go, because as you are well aware, making love draws people closer together.

Making love strengthens that special emotional relationship of intimacy that is not created in any other way I know of.

It draws you very close together emotionally and, I hope, mentally and physically and especially spiritually.

I know you can do it!

Believe and achieve!

I am telling you right now, if you will get your rear in gear, remember:

A SUPER SPIRIT
+
A SUPER MIND
+
A SUPER ATTITUDE
+
A SUPER BODY = SUPER SEX!!

Super Endless Energy

I don't know how your energy is right now, but I'll tell you one thing, if you'll follow my program of Super Fitness, you are going to have endless energy!

By endless energy I mean that you will have so much energy that you will feel like jumping and springing and almost, literally flying!

This great feeling comes when you are Super Fit and:

1. Trim in body weight.
2. When you are super-nourished.
3. When you have been exercising regularly and vigorously.
4. When you have exciting challenges!
5. When you are turned on!

One of the keys to this program of endless energy is, naturally, to be trim, because when you're running around with that extra five, or 10, or 20 pounds, it's holding you down!

To lose weight, increase your physical activity and eat less. For added nutritional insurance take Super Pacs, natural concentrated food supplements.

Walk, run, exercise, play tennis, and so forth.

At first it's hard to increase your physical activity, but, believe me, it gets easier and easier and easier and easier!

So, to have endless energy I want you to increase your physical activity by walking, jogging (if appropriate for your age), running, tennis, swimming, golf and by running in place and jumping jacks and exercise at a health spa at least twice a week.

If you want endless energy, lose weight by following my nutritional tips.

To repeat, my formula for endless energy is:

1. Lose weight by following the nutritional commandments.

2. Exercise daily, any form of physical activity.

Take your photograph and measurements and set goals, as outlined in this book.

Envision in your mind how you are going to look.

Keep enthused and keep working towards your goal of how many pounds you want to lose.

By combining these steps of losing weight and increasing your physical activity, and keeping highly motivated, your energy will GROW EACH DAY until you hit that state which I call ENDLESS ENERGY.

That is when you feel like jumping and doing things because you feel light and springy!

You can do it!

No matter how overweight you are, no matter how logy you are, you can always improve, lose weight and gain energy!

This is the truth.

No shots, pills, surgery, uppers, downers, inners, outers are needed.

This is it!

The truth!

It does involve a certain amount of discipline and hard work, but I'll tell you one thing, it gets easier and easier.

So, that's the price we have to pay for endless energy.

And, remember, I'm only going to tell you the truth.

I am not going to deceive you one bit.

This is the truth and if you will increase your physical activity and follow the nutritional commandments and keep your goal of how much you want to lose envisioned in your mind, you are going to be bouncing along in life instead of dragging along in life.

Super Stress

Most people react to super stress by over-smoking, over-drinking and over-eating.

This reaction to super stress is destructive to the body because of the nicotine in cigarettes, the alcohol in the liquor and the increased stress upon the digestive system from eating too much food, plus the increased stress upon the body to carry around the extra fat.

Sounds simple and logical doesn't it?

But you probably never thought of it that way before. Did you?

My advice to cope with and conquer super stress is:

1. Increase your spiritual life more than ever.

2. Work twice as hard at keeping a super pleasing positive attitude toward your stressful situation and life in general.

3. Greatly increase your physical activity, especially super concentrated physical activity, which I like to call exercise.

Without commenting further on points 1, 2, and 3, I would like to tell you about the super benefits of exercise during stress.

Dr. Menninger of the world famous Menninger Clinic stated that "Exercise is nature's tranquilizer."

The benefits of concentrated physical activity in combatting stress, tension, nervousness are almost miraculous!

1. You can feel the sedative effects of exercise throughout your body almost immediately.

2. Tense muscles contracting during exercise achieve a greater degree of relaxation according to scientific experiments.

3. Circulation is increased, increasing the flow of blood and essential nutrients to all parts of your body — your brain, your internal organs and body tissues.

4. Your nervous system is both tranquilized and prepared for positive action owing to a sympathetic response of the body to exercise.

5. You mental attitude improves because tension is relieved and the chain of stressful negative thoughts are interrupted.

6. The strength and endurance of your muscular system is increased, making you physically able to triumph over your problems.

The point is, exercise will strengthen your spirit, mind, attitude and body because all are ONE!

The stronger you are, the weaker the stress and the easier for you to conquer it.

Remember, TRANQUILIZE WITH EXERCISE!

Super High Naturally

I'm going to tell you how to get high naturally!

How to get turned on without pot, drugs, uppers, downers or drinking.

I am going to tell you how to get a really high feeling.

How to get super duper positively high naturally.

Also how to have a positive attitude and feel as if you can do anything in the world.

And it works!

Step number one: Get into your mind and contemplate on having pleasant positive thoughts.

Now take a protein drink and some natural food supplements.

One hour later, start some type of physical activity.

Take a long walk.

Swim or exercise to music.

Sweat, get active and contract all the muscles in your body.

Get that body stimulated!

While you're exercising, your blood vessels will dilate.

It promotes the assimilation of protein, vitamins and minerals and all the other concentrated SUPER FOODS into your body.

YOU really get high and it's healthy!

You get a tremendously high feeling. The only thing that I can say is, it works!

You are combining pleasant thoughts which are bombarding your mind with the highly concentrated nutritious food so you become naturally high!

There are over 20 grams of protein in each ounce of super quality protein powder and when you add an egg, that makes another six grams.

If you have it with milk, that's another six grams.

So you've got over 30 grams of protein.

If you eat junky food, you feel junky.

If you eat something that's really too sweet, you get a sick feeling within your body.

On the other hand, when you drink a fresh SUPER protein drink with a couple of strawberries it provides vital nutrition for your body.

By combining SUPER food, SUPER thoughts plus SUPER physical activity, you EARN the high feeling.

You will feel SUPER.

I performed some tremendous feats of endurance and stamina which I will never forget during one of my SUPER NATURAL HIGH states.

You'll take those uppers and downers and throw them away!

You'll take the alcohol and toss it out the window!

You won't need artificial stimulants for confidence.

You will get a super high NATURALLY!

Just think, you can do this the rest of your life.

You can enjoy this super high.

When you do this and experience it, write me a letter and tell me about it because it will give me a great deal of satisfaction.

GET HIGH NATURALLY!

Remember: SUPER THOUGHTS + SUPER FOOD + SUPER PHYSICAL ACTIVITY = SUPER HIGH that money cannot buy!

Vacations make you victorious!

Many eminent doctors claim that over 80% of all illnesses are psychosomatic.

I agree with them and probably would put the figure even higher.

Your mind controls your body and if your mind has thoughts of fear, hate, jealousy, rage, lack of security and money worries, all that stress is going to affect your body.

It can lead to ulcers, colitis, skin problems, eye problems and a host of other psychosomatic symptoms.

When you take a vacation and remove yourself from your immediate environment, you often can't remember your problems.

All those problems that loomed so terrifying in your daily routine are hard to remember when you are on vacation.

In fresh surroundings you develop a fresh attitude toward your troubles and allow your self to step back and examine them anew.

Solutions seem to pop into your mind from nowhere!

That's why part of my formula for SUPER FITNESS is to take frequent, short vacations.

Go away someplace for two or three days or just get away over the weekend.

As far as I'm concerned, a vacation every three months is a necessity.

If you can go to the mountains or the seashore, fine; but if you can't afford to get that far away, check into a nearby hotel for a couple of days.

Change your environment!

You'll be amazed to see what it will do to help you unwind and put your problems in the proper perspective.

When you are in the same environment all the time it becomes toxic — poisonous to your mental attitude.

When you get out among the trees and Mother Nature's masterworks, your perspective changes.

Nature didn't build buildings, lay down freeways or install telephones.

Man wasn't meant to live in a concrete jungle.

Man was meant to live among nature.

We humans only have ourselves to blame when we isolate Mother Nature from our lives.

You should get as much fun as possible out of life.

However, it must be in balance with other things.

As your physical nutrition should be balanced so should your mental nutrition.

Work, Fun. Fun . . . Work.

Balance your spiritual life.

There are upper activities and there are downer activities.

Have a hobby!

A hobby is something that you engage in aside from the necessity of earning a living.

The dictionary defines a hobby as an activity that a person chooses to do in his spare time.

Having a hobby is essential for your mental and emotional fitness.

It relieves your mind from the stress of work and it helps maintain balance in your life.

Super vacation and Super fun in your life are but part of the balance needed to achieve SUPER FITNESS.

Money to me is a reward for service.

The more you give, the more you receive.

It is extremely important to have a healthy realistic philosophy about money.

Some people think you have to steal or cheat or lie in order to have it.

No lasting foundation of wealth is based upon falsehood.

The more you sow, the more you reap, says the Bible.

The limit of the money you can earn is directly proportionate to the limits of your thinking and your actions.

Who is to say that if you are earning $500.00 a month that you can't earn $1,000 instead?

Or $2,000 a month?

Or $5,000 or $10,000 or even $50,000 a month?

These are not merely words.

What I am telling you can be translated into reality.

There are no limits to how much you can earn.

The only limits are those you place on yourself.

Set goals for yourself, a monthly goal, a yearly goal and a long range goal of about five years into the future.

Keep your mind open because just one new idea based upon your interests and your abilities can change your financial foundation.

Especially, if you have the courage to act upon that idea.

It happened in my life, and it can happen in yours.

Remember, you receive in relation to what you give.

Follow the principles of Super Success outlined later in this chapter. These principles have evolved from the Bible, from the teachings of Napoleon Hill and scores of other books, magazines and newspaper articles.

I've added some of my own thoughts and interpretations. However, they are principles based upon thousands of hours of research.

Follow these principles of success and you too can earn super money.

a. You can if you think you can.
b. Set your goal and grow each day in every way.
c. Be fair, do not take advantage of others. If you do, you'll be burning your bridges behind you.
d. Go the extra mile.
e. Learn from others.
f. Be persistent.
g. Have courage.
h. Do what you know and feel inside to be right, and your rewards will surely follow.

Whatever you are doing to build your foundation of Super Money, it must be based upon the TRUTH.

If it isn't, your entire structure will crumble and you'll have to start all over again.

With truth as your foundation, and desire as your inspiration, write on paper the goal you wish to achieve.

Write down the specific amount of time and list the specific services that you are going to render to others.

Read your written statement to yourself each morning when you arise and each evening before retiring.

Do this for 31 days and it will automatically put your mind in gear thinking of ways to earn more money, how to improve your present job and how you can render more efficient service.

Before you can earn Super Money, you must develop your Super Mind, your Super Attitude, and your SUPER FITNESS.

This will give you the energy, stamina and endurance you'll need plus the SUPER SPIRIT to give you an everlasting foundation of strength.

You'll need all this in reserve when you run into difficulties and when problems seem hopeless.

With your new life nothing will be hopeless!

Please note that every area of your life including Super Money is interrelated to your total self and Super Money can only be achieved if you are strong and balanced in all areas of your life.

There was a time in my life, in my last year of high school and first year of college, when I thought having money was sinful.

When I heard people talking about money, I thought they were almost evil.

Of course, this was an immature attitude.

The more mature attitude appeared when I realized that money came from service to others — supplying something that other people needed.

It showed me that the amount of prosperity nature creates for a person is in direct proportion to what that person does.

So consider money a reward for your actions.

Do nothing and you'll have nothing.

If you work hard and render the maximum quality and quantity of service to others, you'll earn Super Money and it will be the natural result of your efforts.

When it comes down to the bottom line, Super People earn SUPER MONEY!

Super Natural Beauty

There is no substitute for natural beauty.

Beauty comes from within.

If you are thinking pleasant positive thoughts regularly, if you are enjoying super physical activities and eating super foods, you're going to have super natural beauty.

The increased circulation from the exercises will give you a new younger look.

There is a certain vibrancy about a person who is active physically and mentally.

They emit strong positive vibrations bordering on charisma.

I can spot this type of person in a second.

It takes about the same second to spot the person who is trying to buy beauty by applying powders, creams, salves and all types of concoctions all over their bodies.

You can't buy beauty in a bottle!

Can you imagine a man kissing your skin, but really kissing a heavy layer of powder and cream and paint.

He can taste the difference!

No man wants to eat a bunch of cosmetics.

If you follow my philosophy of living, you'll be a super natural beauty and you won't have to watch your husband's or your boyfriend's face after he kisses a mouthful of greasy powder.

You'll really be "kissable" in every sense of the word.

If you want to highlight your natural beauty, there are natural cosmetics that you can use.

There are papaya and strawberry and other natural source cosmetics without coal tar derivatives.

Soaps, perfumes and colognes are also being made from natural elements.

There is no substitute for a natural vibrant complexion and the super glow of health.

Some of the greatest beauties that I know wear no cosmetics whatsoever.

They eat super foods, they engage in super activities and have super attitudes.

Remember, money cannot buy beauty.

A combination of a super spirit, super thoughts, super attitude, super physical activity and super nutrition will reward you with SUPER BEAUTY which will attract men and turn them on until the day you die!

Super Appearance

If you are ashamed of your appearance, it will naturally affect your mind, your emotions, your attitude about yourself and then your life.

You will not want to go to certain social events.

You won't want to go to the beach in the summer.

You won't be able to wear the latest fashions.

When mini-skirts came out if you had big sloppy fat thighs you would not wear them.

If you have a trim waistline, you'll be proud to show it off instead of hiding your "potbelly!"

Instead of covering yourself from the eyes of others with muu-muu dresses (fat men try to hide in large open shirts), you'll be able to show off your waistline, you'll be able to wear the latest fashions and you'll have that trim, vigorous healthy look that is admired by everyone.

You'll look and feel like a winner.

You will be a winner!

You have to be victorious over YOU.

You can't look super if you don't feel good and you won't feel good if you look lousy.

Remember, your appearance helps to determine the quality of your life.

Think about that for awhile.

Keep your body in super shape.

Let your hair grow out the way you want it.

Take care of your skin, your fingernails and your face.

Wear the latest style clothes.

You don't have to keep up with every fashion and obviously all the new styles aren't for you.

By changing the way you dress, you also change your attitude toward new people and places.

I had a college professor who wore the same suit every day for the entire four years I went to college.

It was unbelievable.

He was archaic.

He lived in an extremely small niche in the world and refused to budge from it.

You want to live in the world, not a niche.

Are you ashamed of your appearance?

Are you proud of your appearance?

If you are proud of it, congratulations!

Make your good looks even better by super food, super exercise and a super pleasing positive mental attitude.

If you are ashamed of your appearance, take a pencil and turn to the page at the end of this book marked "My Personal Ten Commandments for My Super New Life."

Write your resolutions to transform your appearance starting TODAY!

On second thought, a pencil can be erased. Write it down in INK so it will be there every time you open this book!

ENGRAVE your resolutions in your mind.

IMAGINE in your mind your super new appearance.

Now start to transform yourself into your new image.

See yourself daily in your mind looking SUPER!

Hold the new image of yourself in your mind as frequently as possible, at least 15 minutes a day.

This will inspire you to have the discipline and guts and determination to help you transform your appearance and your life into one which can only be described as SUPER!

Below I have listed my personal principles of success. The principles have been acquired over the years from many experiences and extensive reading, especially from the books of Napoleon Hill.

By success, I don't mean just earning a lot of money.

Success is the progressive realization of your goals in life, WHATEVER they may be.

PRINCIPLE NO. 1, POSITIVE THOUGHTS + POSITIVE ACTION

POSITIVE THOUGHTS, followed by POSITIVE ACTION equals success.

There is a saying "Good intentions sometime pave the way to hell."

In this case, with good intentions, positive thoughts plus positive action, you will have success!

PRINCIPLE NO. 2, A BURNING DESIRE

You need a BURNING DESIRE to reach your goals in life.

If you have the attitude maybe I'll do this or maybe I'll do that, you're not going to accomplish anything.

If you're really not turned on or excited, you won't accomplish your goals.

If you want to be the best housewife, the best career person, the best lover, or the best businessman; you must have a burning desire and the amount that you desire will determine the quality of your results.

You must get TURNED ON, EXCITED, STIMULATED AND AGITATED.

You can help build your burning desire by having pictures of what you want.

For instance, if you want a new car — go to a car agency and get a picture.

Frame it in a gold frame.

Put it in your bed or bathroom. Put it someplace where you can see it every day.

Seeing that picture will help you obtain a burning desire.

If you can get a visual aid of whatever it is that you desire and you can see it, this will help stimulate you.

Keep records of your accomplishments.

If you're saving money, look at your bank book and as you see it growing, you'll get excited!

You need visual stimuli to increase your desire.

Think about your goal or what you want to become for five minutes a day or five minutes twice a day.

BUILD YOUR DESIRE!

BUILDING YOUR DESIRE PUTS THE FIRE INSIDE YOU THAT'S GOING TO TURN YOU ON AND KEEP YOU GOING!

PRINCIPLE NO. 3, HAVE A DEFINITE PURPOSE

If you don't know exactly what you want to do, you're not going to do it!

If you don't know what you want to be, STOP and figure it out.

Figure out where you're going!

You don't want your life to be like a ship without a course going around and around in circles.

GET A GOAL, find out at which port you will dock your ship!

MAKE A DECISION AND STICK TO IT!

Get a definite purpose in life. Unfortunately, most people go through life without any special desire.

There are three types of people:

There are people who think they know everything.

There are people who don't know what they think.

Then there are people who don't think in the first place.

GET YOUR MIND IN GEAR!

There are people who cause problems and there are people who solve problems.

GET A DEFINITE PURPOSE IN LIFE AND WRITE IT DOWN. Have it engraved on a piece of wood or perhaps make a drawing of your purpose in life.

My purpose in life is to become the greatest Fitness Crusader in the history of the world.

I have to repeat this to myself constantly.

You must continually keep in your mind what your definite purpose and goal in life is.

Remember, YOU BECOME WHAT YOU THINK ABOUT! As it says in the Bible,

"As ye think in your heart, so ye become."

PRINCIPLE NO. 4, THE MASTER MIND PRINCIPLE

To be SUPER SUCCESSFUL in life, you must apply the master mind principle.

You must learn from and with other people, other MINDS.

There is no single person who knows all the answers.

I learn and you learn from the people we associate with, from what we read, what we think and what we do.

Remember, if you go to bed with dogs, you wake up with fleas!

Try to associate with constructive people who will contribute to your brain and contribute to your thoughts.

The master mind principle means that an EXTRA SUPER MIND is created when you share your thoughts with other minds.

You might call it, FANTASTIC FEEDBACK!

If you're good at math, perhaps you need to associate with people who are more artistic.

An engineer may need a financier for an associate.

No one person knows everything.

You learn from everybody!

You should have meetings with members of your master-mind group regularly.

I have meetings with certain people once a week.

It helps me reach my goals.

It helps make life more interesting when you share your mind with other people.

The mastermind principle teaches you that SUPER SUCCESS in life comes from HARMONIOUS MENTAL and PHYSICAL EFFORT with other human beings.

PRINCIPLE NO. 5, FAITH

Without FAITH, life is hopeless!

No matter what you're doing, you must have FAITH!

Without FAITH you will NEVER become a SUPER SUCCESS in life.

Worship as you wish, but worship. That's part of my philosophy, but you need faith in the creator and faith in YOURSELF!

SUPER FAITH IS PART OF THE KEY TO YOUR SUPER SUCCESS!

PRINCIPLE NO. 6, A PLEASING PERSONALITY

If you go around insulting people, continually being mean, being a sour apple, you won't be a SUPER SUCCESS, no matter what your goal may be.

You may be successful by your own definition, by having earned a substantial amount of money, but you'll never be a success by my definition or the definition of most people because you'll be lonely.

You won't have friends.

No one wants to be around a sour, negative or destructive person.

You want to be pleasant!

A pleasing personality is a vital part of your formula for SUPER SUCCESS.

PRINCIPLE NO. 7, GOING THE EXTRA MILE

Develop the habit of always doing MORE work than you are paid for.

If your job calls for you to work 40 hours a week and it becomes necessary to work 50 or 60, go that EXTRA MILE.

This is the person who will get the promotions.

This is the person who is given bonuses.

I am constantly extending myself.

For instance, one night I drove an extra 40 miles to see someone who needed help on a problem.

I didn't see any benefit in it for myself, but I did it anyway.

I did it because I get satisfaction from helping people.

Fortunately, anytime you do something for others it bounces back at YOU.

You may not receive the return benefits for one or two years or even ten years, but going that extra mile allows you to give a little more than is required of yourself and you receive the benefits tenfold, and not always from the same source.

The more you put into each exercise the more benefit you get out of it. The better you practice SUPER NUTRITION, the greater the benefits to your SUPER FITNESS. Remember, "As ye sow, so shall ye reap!"

PRINCIPLE NO. 8, INITIATIVE

Initiative is getting your REAR IN GEAR!

If you're sitting around waiting for someone else to get something going — it will NEVER get started.

You have got to have initiative.

You have to overcome stagnation.

When water stagnates it can't circulate like a rippling trickling brook, it gets sick!

It's the same with your mind.

If it's stagnant, it starts backing up and gets filled with poisonous thoughts.

It's the same with food, if it isn't digested, or eliminated, it actually pollutes your body.

You must get turned on. IT'S NOT EASY, BUT YOU CAN DO IT! So develop SUPER INITIATIVE, GET YOUR REAR IN GEAR!

PRINCIPLE NO. 9, SELF-DISCIPLINE

Either you discipline yourself or you will be disciplined by others.

When the people of a Nation become weak, fat and lazy, eventually they will be controlled by conquerors.

It may take five, ten or twenty years or fifty or a hundred years, but the Roman empire is a wondrous example of losing self discipline and losing your freedom.

So, you must have discipline because if you don't, you'll be controlled by others and you will lose a certain part of your freedom.

If you have self discipline, you can earn more money and this money can give you freedom.

If you plug along on some average job because you need a pay check each month from some boss, you're giving a certain amount of freedom up for that pay check.

If you have the discipline to set and reach your goals and grow to do things, and learn not to be so dependent on others, you have gained freedom.

SELF DISCIPLINE is one of the SUPER KEYS to life.

You can't do ten things at once.

You can't even do two things at once successfully.

You must CONCENTRATE.

If you're going to cook, don't read the paper or do a number of other things at the same time.

Concentrate on your creation.

Have a vision in your mind of how it will taste.

Put the seasoning in at the right time. Control the temperature perfectly.

If you're painting a picture, don't read a book at the same time.

If you're going to paint you have to concentrate on it.

If you're reading, cut out distractions and concentrate!

Concentrate on everything that you do.

Concentration is one of the most important principles of success.

If you don't concentrate, you're not going to be 100% successful in what you're doing.

You'll be 90% or 80% or maybe just 40%.

The percentage of successful completion of anything will depend a great deal upon your CONCENTRATION.

PRINCIPLE NO. 11, ENTHUSIASM

The word enthusiasm comes from theos, which means Godlike in Greek.

Enthusiasm is a wondrous ingredient.

It ignites life.

Enthusiasm makes you feel that life is worthwhile.

Enthusiasm makes hard work become easy.

Enthusiasm is contagious, it fills you with spirit.

Enthusiasm turns everyone on.

Enthusiasm makes a rainy day sunny.

EVERYBODY LIKES AN ENTHUSIASTIC PERSON!
Enthusiasm makes your work play!

It helps you reach your goals!

If you dislike something, don't have it as your goal.

My formula to choose your vocation is: INTEREST + ABILITIES = VOCATION.

When you take your interest and your abilities and add them together, this leads to enthusiasm because you are doing things which you enjoy.

If you don't like your work, get a different job!

You don't have to stay in the same job.

If you are married to the wrong mate, get a new one!

If you're not enthusiastic about your mate, you have a problem.

Enthusiasm is a magic ingredient for your success.

PRINCIPLE NO. 12, IMAGINATION

Imagination will help you earn a SUPER home, SUPER clothes, a SUPER hairdo, make you a SUPER lover and give you imagination for your work.

You'll get new ideas on how to improve the way you're working, maybe think of an idea that could revolutionize your job or your life!

Spend a little time each day expanding your imagination.

I personally know, the harder you work, the better your imagination becomes.

Your brain is like a computer to some extent, and the more facts and experience you fill your brain with, the better your imagination will become.

Work hard on stimulating your imagination.

Have as a goal the development of a SUPER imagination.

You should always learn from adversity.

Many people give up easily. They slip once and they are finished.

No successful person has been successful in everything all the time!

There will ALWAYS be some adversity.

There will ALWAYS be some problems!

You'll have friends who will disappoint you at times, but don't desert them for a little human error because NOBODY IS PERFECT!

When the going gets tough, THE TOUGH GET GOING.

WINNERS NEVER QUIT AND QUITTERS NEVER WIN.

Keep thinking positive and keep yourself enthused.

Adversity destroys many people, but it also CREATES winners.

If you lose the first time, simply say; alright, I'm going to get going and this time I will WIN.

The world's greatest doers didn't always win the first time.

Roger Bannister almost gave up running until he finally got mad at himself and broke the four minute mile.

How many people have marriages that end up in divorce?

If they have small minds, they will give up and say things like; marriage is for the birds, or all women are out for your money or all men are just out for your body.

When people form adverse generalizations, they get sour in life, crawl into holes like moles and rot away their life.

All of us know people like this.

Learn from adversity.

Don't make the same mistake twice.

Triumph over your defeats.

Learn from your defeats.

Never give in to any situation that violates good sense and justice.

Winston Churchill, one of the greatest leaders in the history of mankind is a great example.

When England was facing its bleakest days and the Germans were dropping rockets on England — things were looking gloomy and it seemed that England would be conquered — Winston Churchill by the strength of his enthusiasm, spirit and fortitude inspired the country to triumph.

He wrote, in one of his most famous speeches, "Never give in!"

The truth is, you CAN'T give in.

If you give in, you will sink lower and lower in life.

Many sections of proverbs in the Bible refer to the pit: the depthless pit in which people can fall when they lose their self-respect or self-confidence.

They lose their meaning to life.

They've given up in life.

Many people even commit suicide.

Did you ever stop to think of suicide as just plain giving up in life?

You CAN win.

You WILL triumph over your adversities.

Think of every adversity as an OPPORTUNITY and you will learn to turn your defeats into TRIUMPHS.

PRINCIPLE NO. 14, BUDGETING OF TIME

To be successful you must budget your time.

The only limited factor you have in life is your time.

Every minute of your life is ticking away, never to come back.

Once it's gone, it's GONE!

Many people waste their time by lying around doing nothing.

Small talk is very good and very healthy to a certain degree.

Many people allow others to waste a huge amount of their time.

Allow a certain amount of time to play, to work, enjoy friends, for worship, for expansion of your mind.

But budget your time or it will tick away and one day you'll say, "WHERE DID MY LIFE GO?"

If this happens, you'll have one person to blame, YOURSELF!

PRINCIPLE NO. 15, ACCURATE THINKING

Accurate thinking.

Try to separate your fantasies from the facts.

Try to think accurately.

Try to let your emotions help you enjoy life and all the beauty in life.

Try to think clearly and logically.

Ask yourself, am I spending more than I'm earning?

Are you earning more than you are spending?

Get the numbers, add them up.

GET THE FACTS.

Make your decisions based on facts not fantasies.

Don't make important decisions in a whirlwind of emotions.

THINK ACCURATELY.

Use your brain. This incredible powerful organ is often neglected.

ACCURATE THINKING IS ESSENTIAL FOR SUPER LIVING!

PRINCIPLE NO. 16, VIGOROUS EMOTIONAL SPIRITUAL, MENTAL AND PHYSICAL HEALTH

The next principle is SUPER emotional, spiritual, mental and physical health.

Super spiritual, mental and physical health can be yours if you practice every thing listed in this chapter.

Recently, a world renowned billionaire died.

He was worth literally billions of dollars, but the second he lost his health, his wealth became worthless.

HEALTH IS WEALTH!

One of our goals in Super Fitness is Super Health!

This is one of the cornerstones of life because without health, not much else matters.

PRINCIPLE NO. 17, COOPERATION!

We all need cooperation.

You need the cooperation of people.

You need friends.

No single person can do everything by himself.

You get this from having a pleasing attitude.

By giving!

By serving!

By helping people.

When you help others, they will help you.

If you are only a taker, they will catch on quick enough.

You'll find when you call them, they will be in a rush, or they'll be just leaving, or perhaps they don't want to talk to you at all.

You need cooperation of others working together in harmony.

You must work in SUPER HARMONY or you won't be SUPER SUCCESSFUL.

This last principle will automatically come to you when you have effected all the other principles.

It's sort of a sixth sense.

It's based upon love and faith.

When you have practiced all the other principles and you're working hard, giving and growing, studying and learning, and also going that extra mile, you seem to get divine guidance.

The answers to your questions seem to come automatically.

You seem to be steered by a super power!

Some of you have experienced it and know exactly what I'm talking about.

If you haven't experienced it, you will if you practice all the other principles of success.

All I can say is, there are some things in life that are more miraculous than words can ever explain.

How many stars are there in the sky?

How big are they?

How high does the sky go?

Where does it end?

When did time begin? When will it end?

Why was man born?

What happens after death?

Life is more wondrous than you'll ever know and the sixth sense, the divine guidance of your life will come if you practice the other principles of success.

Remember, success is not just money, it's being successful in doing your thing.

Follow these SUPER principles of success and turn your dreams into reality.

YOU CAN DO IT. YOU ARE DOING IT, as of this moment.

CONGRATULATIONS on your SUPER SUCCESS!

Personal Messages To Senior Citizens, Homemakers, Youth

Senior Citizens

Unfortunately, many senior citizens die within one year after retirement.

Senior citizens must have a goal in life also, whether it is a hobby or a part-time job or service to others. A goal in life, in this case, is a matter of life or death.

If you are on a tight budget do not eliminate the essential foods to save money.

Many senior citizens suffer from malnutrition in an attempt to buy the cheapest and therefore, the lowest quality food. Make sure you take your food supplements. Make sure you have a sufficient protein intake. Make sure you have fresh fruits and vegetables. Make sure you have enough roughage, such as ALL-BRAN, for healthy elimination.

Have regular physical activities.

Don't just lie around watching television or sitting in the sun with a shawl.

There are many things you can do to get out of that rut of non-physical activity.

Walking, I think, is the number one exercise for senior citizens.

Walking is a natural body refreshener and tremendous for circulation.

It keeps your joints mobile and flexible.

When I was a physical therapist doing all the therapy in a convalescent hospital for 250 senior citizens whose average age was about 75, I treated hundreds of people with "frozen" knees.

These people had been sitting for so long that they couldn't move their legs. I worked with people with "frozen" elbows. They couldn't bend their arms.

I worked with people who had "frozen" shoulders and "frozen" fingers. After a joint is "frozen," especially when one gets older, it is extremely difficult to make it mobile again.

So put all your joints into motion daily.

This is very important.

Raise your arms over your head, bend your arms, make circles with your arms, in a circle, open and close your fingers. Take warm baths.

Be sure to keep those joints mobile.

The senior citizen should also have a hobby.

It's a matter of life and death also. Something that involves some reading, some physical movement and some contact with others who enjoy the same.

If you're not married get a girl friend!

To hell with what people might say. Get a girl friend (or a boy friend) and start stepping out and going places together.

Again, it's a matter of survival.

As long as you maintain a goal in life and you're active physically and mentally, life is going to be SUPER. But the second you start becoming inactive and moping around and feeling sorry for yourself, you're committing SUICIDE.

I also strongly recommend that you do not become isolated and shut others out of your life.

No one man is an island . . . and no woman is either! EVERYBODY NEEDS PEOPLE.

We learn from other people.

We are inspired by other people.

When you help other people, you receive satisfaction because those people turn around and help you! Try to associate with a group of people who are younger than yourself or young thinking senior citizens.

If you are in a convalescent hospital there is nothing that says you have to lie in bed and rot.

If you stay in that bed you WILL ROT!

THE BED IS YOUR #1 ENEMY!
THE CHAIR IS YOUR #2 ENEMY!
WALKING IS YOUR #1 FRIEND!

Stay away from your #1 and your #2 enemy, but make close ties with your #1 friend. If you don't want your joints to "freeze," MOVE THEM.

Have lots of friends.

When you are a senior citizen, friends can mean the difference between a super life and a living death.

Most health spas have a special rate for senior citizens and I recommend spas because most have a 105-degree therapy pool which can do wonders for your circulation.

It's a great place to exercise your joints to keep them limber.

A spa is both a social and a therapeutic center under one roof.

If you are a senior citizen you know that an ounce of prevention in terms of your physical health is worth a pound of cure.

Homemakers

I definitely believe that being a homemaker is the world's hardest profession.

The homemaker is confined to one environment a great deal of the time, which can become extremely stagnant and toxic if not varied with outside interests and friends.

The homemaker is expected to clean up after the rest of the family, prepare the meals and is frequently regarded as a servant for the rest of the family.

The routine of homemaking can become extremely monotonous.

I recommend the homemaker start off the day the SUPER FITNESS way!

One should start with prayer and meditation.
Next, do exercises.

Follow this by a nourishing breakfast that includes a protein drink and natural food supplements.

She should also read at least 30 minutes daily, including some inspirational reading to give her the enthusiasm to motivate the rest of her family.

The homemaker should definitely have activities that take her out of the house on a regular basis.

It should be something she looks forward to.

She should have interesting and stimulating friends who are positive influences in her life.

She should stay away from people who are continually telling her all their problems, dragging her down and literally sucking her life-energy.

I recommend she avoid the chain smokers and the habitual coffee drinkers. Remember, you become a product of your environment.

She should be sure to accentuate the positive and eliminate the negative.

If you are a homemaker and feel that you are in a rut, then join some friends in dancing lessons, horseback riding, hiking or some other physical activity.

I recommend a health club or spa where you can do your exercises regularly, where you can receive inspiration, nutritional information, where you can share activities with other homemakers.

Other excellent activities are swimming, golf and bicycle riding.

Having pleasant company makes fitness fun.

Remember: When you are uptight, tranquilize with exercise!

Exercise is nature's tranquilizer.

I'd also like to see you have a vegetable garden of your own. It takes very little space to grow your own vegetables and since you won't spray them with DDT you won't be feeding your family poison-coated food.

I have a garden about 15 x 20 feet. I grow tomatoes, string beans, squash, celery and scrumptious eggplant.

Fresh home grown food is wonderful for your loved ones and is also an excellent hobby for you and the entire family.

A main point for homemakers is, get out of your rut!

Remember that the only difference between a rut and a grave is the depth!

It's up to you to be victorious over yourself, your procrastinations, your fears, your doubts, your stagnation.

If you want to be a wise wife, I definitely recommend that you invest at least one hour each day in yourself.

In your appearance!

In your beauty!

You want to be attractive and stimulating to your mate and you don't want him concentrating on his secretary or the girls in the office.

If you neglect your body, if you don't keep yourself looking alluring, it's your own fault.

So, invest in the most important person in the world: YOURSELF!

Forget all your excuses!

Set a goal of what you want to weigh.

Fill out the weight chart and fitness folder in this book.

Decide what your normal weight should be and then strive to become the most attractive, enthusiastic, pleasant, positive wife in the world.

Make this your goal and reach it!

You CAN do it!

Remember, that homemaking — your profession — is the foundation of humanity!

The knowledge and attitudes of the mother are transferred to her children at the extremely formative ages of one to five, and many psychologists say that the actual personality that remains with the child all through his life is formed at this time.

The homemaker determines the quality of food that nourishes her family.

Never stop searching for ways to improve the nutrition of your family.

Your husband depends upon you for emotional support.

When it looks like everything is going wrong and his business or job is collapsing, you are the one who gives him the hope and the support to keep pushing.

There are times when it looks as if everyone's life is about to collapse around you.

YOU'VE GOT TO BE STRONG!

Many times you are the only person who really cares what happens to your husband.

So, the homemaker is actually the BACKBONE of our entire SOCIETY.

There is the saying: BEHIND EVERY SUCCESSFUL MAN, IS A WISE WOMAN.

It's true.

I'm sure you don't want the woman behind your successful man to be someone else.

Get your rear in gear!

Keep yourself active spiritually, physically and mentally so you can enthuse and encourage your children and your husband, and build a truly SUPER FAMILY!

Youths

The food that the average child eats is both trash and tragic.

Many mothers choose their children's nutrition by whether or not the child wants to have a certain prize in a box!

The mother feels that as long as the child eats something, it's better than nothing.

HOW WRONG SHE IS!

Many mothers poison their children without knowing it.

I have stressed throughout this book that YOU ARE WHAT YOU EAT.

I recommend that no refined sugar of any kind be given to children.

Sugar destroys tooth enamel and creates cavities in growing teeth.

Your children will receive enough natural sugar in the fruits they eat.

You can give them honey, but not in excessive amounts.

Allow no candy that is made from sugar.

Let your children eat dates, figs, raisins, sunflower and pumpkin seeds.

Colas and sodas are loaded with refined white sugar.

Your children should also have a protein drink in the morning, but make sure the protein powder you buy contains no sugar.

Mix an egg in with it or some fresh strawberries or put a banana in it and call it a banana milkshake.

You should flavor the child's protein powder naturally with fresh fruit.

See how wonderful your children will feel and look when they start taking a delicious protein drink.

Be certain that you don't serve your child those foodless foods that have been "shot from guns," "oven baked" and "super enriched" with artificial flavors and coated with sweeteners.

STUDY the section of this book about SUPER NUTRITION.

It applies to children as well as adults.

Stay away from products with preservatives.

Make sure the fruits and vegetables you serve are fresh and free of pesticides.

And don't forget to include cottage cheese, lean meat, fresh poultry and fresh fish in the daily diet.

Naturally, make sure your child gets enough physical activity.

Limit TV time intelligently!

A child must have guidance. You are the parent.

Who is more capable of shaping your child's future?

You with your adult knowledge, or the child with his immature ways?

Up to the age of about 12, children don't have to do any formal exercise.

In my opinion most children get enough exercise before that age through normal playing.

To build your children's self-esteem don't tear them down all the time.

Don't keep harping on how sloppy they are.

Don't keep telling them what losers they are.

Don't poison their mind.

Many parents do this without even knowing it.

Say things in a positive way.

Say "How neat you're going to be when you learn to pick up everything."

Or "You're going to be very smart when you finish reading the book."

Or "With just a little more effort you CAN do it."

Plant the thought in your children's mind that they are going to be successful and that you love them.

Many people are in mental hospitals today because their parents planted negative thoughts in their minds as children.

No flower will grow properly if you keep stomping it back into the earth.

Remember, that you are what you hear, what you think, what you do and what you eat!

If a child is continually hearing how bad he or she is, they will start to believe it and will become bad.

So, when you talk to your child, listen to your own words and evaluate if your lectures are building or destroying your child.

Remember the negativity your parents piled upon you.

Don't do the same thing to YOUR own child.

Build up your children and they will love you and make you proud of them for the rest of your life.

Tear them down continually and they will disappear as soon as they can.

Remember, children follow examples, not words.

If you want your child to have healthy living habits, YOU should have healthy living habits.

If you smoke, your child will see you doing it and want to smoke also.

The same goes for drinking or sloppy dressing or unclean personal habits.

Don't eat junk foods, canned foods or frozen foods because that's what your child will want to eat.

People say that fatness runs in the family.

The only reason it does is usually because it's a habit the children learned from their parents.

SET AN EXAMPLE!

Children follow the leader.

They learn from the actions of their parents and usually reflect their parents outside the home.

If you want SUPER children, be A SUPER parent.

Feed them SUPER FOOD,

give them SUPER activity,

give them SUPER love and

give them SUPER thoughts and attitudes!

Personal Message Regarding
The Cost of Being Sick

It is much easier and less expensive to be Super Fit not Super Sick.

Read the following startling set of statistics.

They are based on insurance company's figures for the year 1974.

(1) The cost per day of an average hospital bed: $110.00
(2) Dollar value of time lost due to sickness in U.S. $7,000,000,000.00
(3) Estimate of money spent on medicines in U.S. $22,500,000,000.00
(4) Number of work time lost due to sickness: 757,000 man years
(5) Estimated number of alcoholics in U.S. 10,000,000
(6) Estimated number heart disease patients in U.S. 125,000,000
(7) Estimated number of cancer victims in U.S. 30,000,000
(8) Estimated number overweight people in U.S. 150,000,000
(9) How many cavities needing fillings in American Teeth: 750,000,000
(10) How many pounds of aspirin swallowed by Americans: 25 million pounds.

People make themselves sick.

People do not get sick.

They do it to themselves.

They make themselves sick from improper living habits.

UNHEALTHY NUTRITION OF THE MIND (THOUGHTS).

UNHEALTHY NUTRITION OF THE BODY (FOOD).

A lack of sufficient physical activity.

Negative destructive attitudes plus inadequate rest adds up to SICKNESS!

A few years ago, Dr. David Stonecypher, a Boston specialist in aging, reported:

"Most people expect their bodies to degenerate automatically with age and develop such frightening diseases such as arthritis, cataracts and heart attacks.

But these diseases are not caused by growing old.

The damage is caused by persistent strain to an organ or to bad nutrition.

There are probably no diseases caused by growing old.

There is nothing about old age that necessitates poor health."

People make themselves sick!

IT'S EASIER AND LESS EXPENSIVE AND MORE FUN TO BE SUPER FIT!

Take Your Choice

SICKNESS	SUPER FITNESS
(1) Feel Bad	(1) Feel Super
(2) Look Sloppy	(2) Look Super
(3) Lack Energy	(3) Super Energy
(4) Lose Desire	(4) Burning Desires
(5) Immobile	(5) Action!
(6) Can't Work	(6) Industrious
(7) Life is a Struggle	(7) Life is a Ball
(8) Dull Mind	(8) Dynamic Mind
(9) Sinking Spirit	(9) Soaring Spirit
(10) Live in a Rut	(10) Live in a World
(11) Problem Oriented	(11) Challenge Oriented
(12) Grumpy Attitude	(12) Pleasant Attitude
(13) Can't Cut the Mustard	(13) Super Sex
(14) Broke	(14) Super Money
(15) Negativity	(15) Positivity

Earn Super Fitness or End Up With

Super Sickness!

As a human being you should grow better each day and in every way: spiritually, mentally, attitude-wise and physically.

If you do not grow, you shrink!

Your wondrous spirit, mind and body constitute the most intricate creations on earth.

Their capacity for development is limitless, as is the healthy joy, yes, even the rapture you can attain from SUPER LIVING.

Exercise your spirit daily, ideally each morning and each evening.

Exercise your miraculous mind.

Control your thoughts and control your destiny on earth.

Develop pleasant, positive attitudes regarding the world you live in.

As Robert Kennedy said, "Dream not how things are, but how they can become."

Reality exists only in your state of mind.

Accentuate the positive and eliminate the negative.

Remember, as I have often stated in this book, THE THOUGHTS YOU ALLOW YOUR MIND TO THINK ARE MORE IMPORTANT THAN THE FOOD YOU EAT.

Even though I am vitally concerned with nutrition of the body, "nutrition of the mind" (thoughts) is even more important.

Use your God-given body daily in as much vigorous physical activity as often as possible, for if you rest too much, YOU'LL RUST!

The human body, unlike a machine, improves with use and regresses with too much rest.

Feed the temple of your soul — your body — with fresh alive foods.

Dead foods do not produce super-alive bodies.

Supplement your diet with natural concentrated super food supplements.

The better you nourish your body the better you will look, feel and be.

Grow daily, in every way, in spirit, mind, attitude and body.

You CAN make your dreams come true!

Life at its most basic level is survival of the fittest, that's why SUPER FITNESS to you and to me means living the wondrous radiant healthy and happy SUPER LIFE we all should seek.

1. Believe and have FAITH.

2. Believe in YOU.

3. Set a personal lifetime goal that excites you.
4. Get your rear in gear and start working to achieve that goal.
5. Follow my plan for, Super Development of:

SPIRIT
MIND
ATTITUDE
BODY

This book is not the last word regarding SUPER FITNESS.

This book represents my first step in recording thoughts which will help you live a SUPER LIFE.

Each day I add to my understanding of SUPER FITNESS and how to attain it and maintain it.

Daily I meet with others in the fitness profession and learn from them.

Daily I read about fitness.

Daily I experiment with my own spirit, mind, attitude and body and grow from each experience.

So it is that you must grow daily in every way in order to strive for your epitome of SUPER FITNESS and SUPER LIVING.

Everything that I learn, experience and understand about body and mind development after this book goes to press will be incorporated in SUPER FITNESS II.

"The glory of kings is to search out a matter."

In this case How To Be Super Fit and how
To Enjoy A Super Life!

So seek and ye shall find YOUR SUPER NEW LIFE!

My Personal 10 Commandments
for My Super New Life

I.

II.

III.

IV.

V.

VI.

VII.

VIII.

IX.

X.

Make a Resolution

Make a resolution to yourself right now to live the SUPER FITNESS way of life.

You owe it to yourself, to your family and your loved ones.

If for some reason you feel you have no loved ones: you will!

By living the SUPER FITNESS way you will attract others to you who are also positive and exciting.
Say to yourself now:
I will think, read, analyze.
Refreshing new thoughts
Upon which to build my wonderful new life.
I will have
A pleasing attitude.
I will see the good in life
And turn everything into an asset.
I will control my mind and my mouth
Eat wisely.
Exercise daily.
I want to be BORN ANEW,
To burst forth with energy and stamina,
Vigor and enthusiasm
And triumph over life itself.
O wonder of wonders,
O meaning of meanings,
O power of powers
May I spread
Joy, health and happiness.
The Super Fitness
Way of Life.

The products mentioned in "Super Fitness" are brand names marketed by the author's company, Super Fitness of America. Similar products, especially those dealing with nutrition, are available under different names in retail outlets.

Super Food™, Super Pac™, Super Belt™, Super Pants™, and Trimex™, mentioned in this book may be ordered by writing:

Super Fitness of America
23650 Hawthorne Boulevard
Torrance, California 90505